Uncorrec *Not for circulation*

Ariadne Then and Now

The Labyrinth and the End of Times

(Third Edition)

With best wishes

Carol Matthews

Carol

NeoPoiesis Press, LLC

2775 Harbor Ave SW, Suite D, Seattle, WA 98126-2138
Inquiries: Info@NeoPoiesisPress.com
NeoPoiesisPress.com

Carol Matthews -
ISBN 979-8-9858336-0-7 (pbk)

1. Aging. 2. Death. 3. Mindfulness I. Matthews, Carol. II. Ariadne Then and Now: The Labyrinth and the End of Times

Library of Congress Control Number: 2022941546

Third Edition

Cover Design: Dale Winslow and Rob Hall

Printed in the United States of America.

This new edition is dedicated to my granddaughter, Charlotte, and to her grandfather, Mike, who walked many labyrinths with her.

I thought of a labyrinth of labyrinths, of one sinuous spreading labyrinth that would encompass the past and future...

—Jorge Luis Borges, *The Garden of Forking Paths*

A labyrinth is a symbolic journey . . . but it is a map we can really walk on, blurring the difference between map and world.

—Rebecca Solnit, *Wanderlust: A History of Walking*

Contents

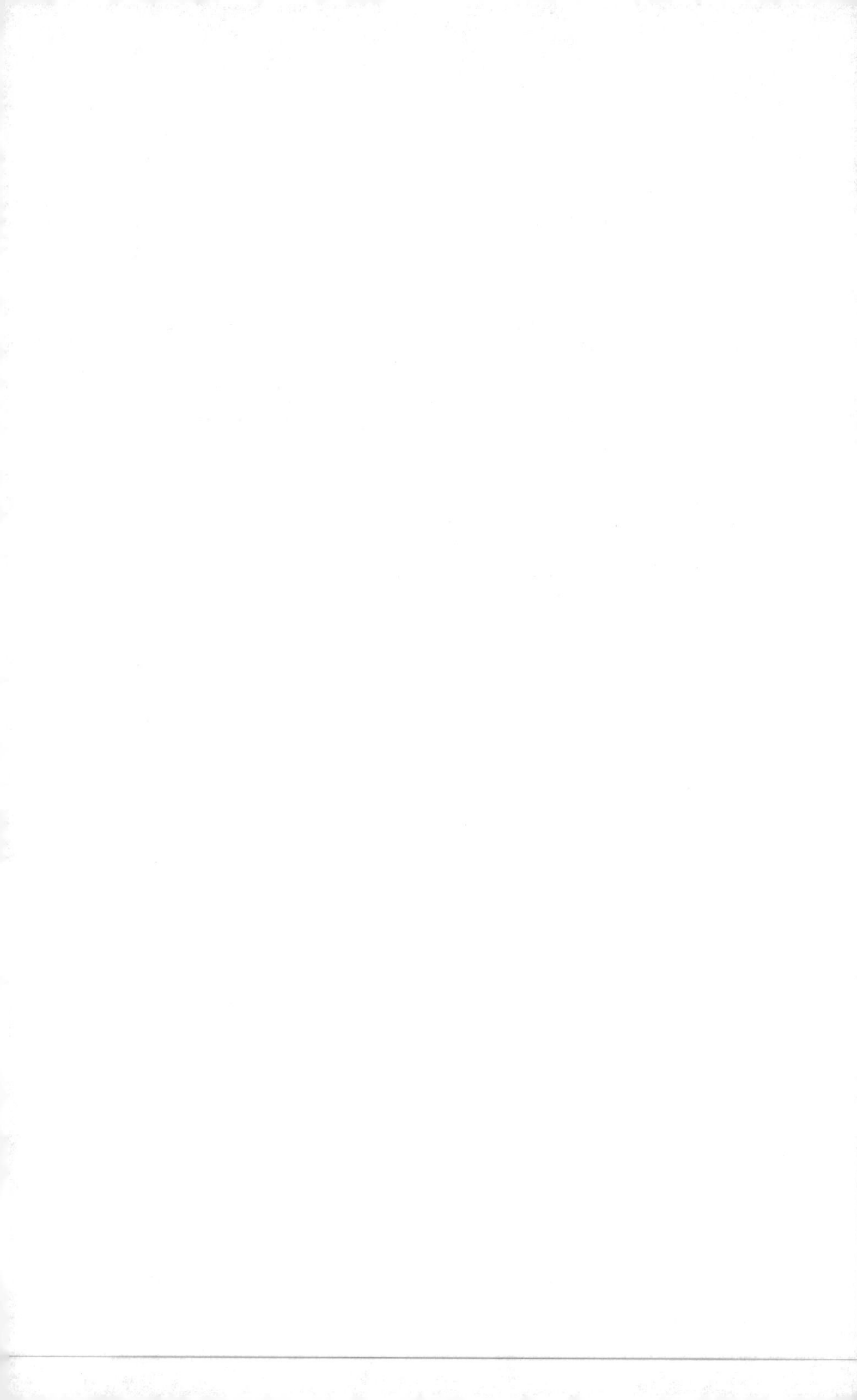

Introduction

Life is a journey, not a destination. This famous quote by Ralph Waldo Emerson expresses the idea that what matters most is the process rather than the product. The trip is not a means to an end—in the end, it is its own end. Life, to say the least, is *trippy*.

The medium is the message, said Marshall McLuhan. The journey is the medium that connects the beginning of the trip to its final destination, but the meaning of the journey is not to be found at either extreme, but in the act of journeying, the act of living. Albert Einstein explained that the universe is not made up of *things*, but rather of *events*. All phenomena are dynamic, unfolding, everchanging. We are all a part of one enormous *happening*, with no fixed point from which to survey our surroundings, instead constantly in motion, so that there all we can know for certain are relations and relationships. Buckminster Fuller dubbed our planet *Spaceship Earth*, and we collectively partake in our world's journey through spacetime in addition to our own, personal travels and travails.

'Tain't What You Do (It's the Way That You Do It) relates the song made famous by Ella Fitzgerald in 1939, a song echoed in a remark by the main character, Jude, in the 2007 Beatles-inspired film, *Across the Universe*: During an exchange that illustrates the generation gap between the baby boomers and their parents, an older family member insists that *what you do defines who you are*, while the younger one disagrees, countering, *who you are defines what you do*. He then turns to Jude and asks if he agrees, to which Jude replies, *surely, it's not what you do, but the way that you do it*. The *way*, the *path*, the *road*, represents a metaphor often used to represent changes over time, transitions, and growth, as well as forms of religious observance and spiritual enlightenment most notably in the concept of the *Tao* or *Dao* and the concomitant system of Taoism.

All roads lead to Rome, or so goes the old adage. Left unsaid is the fact that in antiquity all roads led to Rome because it was the Romans who built them. As a metaphor, however, the saying points to the idea that there are many ways to get to the same destination. In some instances, some may say that there is a *right way* and a *wrong way* to reach our goal, and that some of us have *lost our way* or *found our way*. Still, the underlying concession is that there is always *more than one way* to get to wherever we're going. If life is the journey in question, then the Rome of our roaming is death, the final destination. And yet, and yet, we know that all roads are not the same, that what counts is the way that we arrive at the great leveler at journey's end.

O ye'll tak' the high road, and I'll tak' the low road, goes the chorus of the Scottish song, "The Bonnie Banks o' Loch Lomond," where the low road is premature death suffered by a young soldier. Roads can be high or low, rough or smooth, long or short. And the kind of path we're on is not always clear and visible to us. Sometimes we just have to make our way forward based on nothing more than faith and hope, putting one foot in front of another. McLuhan invoked the metaphor of the rearview mirror in talking about the past, present, and future. We often depict life's journey as if the future is in front of us and the past behind us. But in truth, the future is hidden from view, whereas the past is known to us, open for inspection and introspection. In this sense, we march backwards into the future, always looking at the past, never knowing where we're headed.

The shortest distance between two points is a straight line, or so we learn in grade school. But what we typically aren't told, even when looking at maps, is that this is only true within Euclidean geometry, and only applies to flat surfaces. When it comes to spheres, like our planet, the shortest distance is a curved line, an arc, part of a great circle. And sometimes *going in circles* is exactly the reason for the journey. We speak of *coming full circle*, and *returning to the source*, as journeys may take us someplace new, but also may eventually bring us back home. We refer to a long journey as an *odyssey*, but after all, the Homeric epic, the *Odyssey*, is the story of Odysseus's long and difficult journey home. Baseball too involves a circular path away from home with the hope of returning once again. Joseph Campbell's monomythic hero's journey, and its parallel in rites of passage such as those associated with puberty, involve the hero leaving home, undergoing a series of tests and trials and thereby gaining gifts, and then returning home to use those gifts for the benefit of those who were earlier left behind. It follows, then, that the death has often been framed as a home-coming, a return from whence we came, so that the life is a journey that is circular in nature.

Not all who wander are lost, wrote J.R.R. Tolkien. There is a difference between meandering, or simply taking the scenic route, as opposed to wandering aimlessly. Nomadic tribes are not lost in the wilderness, nor do they travel directionless and without purpose. Rather, they trace pre-ordained routes, following the seasons, migrating in accordance with cyclical changes, returning over and over again to familiar stops along their circuit. The jour-ney is ongoing, never reaching a final destination. And travel is undertaken in accordance with the environment, not as a means of overcoming and taking possession of it.

Slow down, you move too fast, sing Paul Simon and Art Gar-funkel at the start of *The 59th Street Bridge Song*. Speeding up is an attempt to bypass the journey in favor of getting to the destination as quickly as possible, minimizing if not eliminating the experience of traveling. Rapid transit is nothing more than a means to an end. Not being in a hurry, moving at a leisurely pace, rambling and am-bling along, maybe even dawdling at times, prolongs the journey, and allows the traveler to appreciate the trip and, in the words of the old admonition, to *stop and smell the roses*."

The journey, the way we travel, the path we take, its di-rection and its directness, whether straight or circuitous, whether one-way or round trip, whether fast or slow, all are differences that make a difference. And all relate to the labyrinth, the theme and metaphor that guides and informs Carol Matthews in both the content and the style of this memoir and meditation.

We typically think of the term *labyrinth* as a synonym for *maze*, and Matthews is quick to disabuse the reader of such notions. A maze is a puzzle, the challenge being to find the right path among many false and misleading passages. Not so a labyrinth, which is a winding road that takes you deep into its space, and then brings you out again. In a labyrinth, you may not know where you are, or how distant the entrance or exit may be, but the path will al-ways lead you back out eventually. The danger of entering a maze is getting so lost as to never finding your way back out amidst all of the alternative routes available to you. The danger in the labyrinth is in part the threat of its denizens, i.e., the Minotaur, thereby being lost *to* the monstrous other. Alongside the physical danger, there is the psychological danger of giving up hope, of being lost *due to* being overwhelmed by the illusion that there is no exit, that the path has no end point, that you can never find your way out again.

The labyrinth is what Gregory Bateson refers to as a *metapattern*. There is the labyrinth of myth made famous by the story of Ariadne, with whom Matthews engages in imaginary conversations sprinkled throughout the book, and Theseus, and the Minotaur. There are real life labyrinths that can be found throughout the world, open to the public, and Matthews is an experienced labyrinth walker who readily relates the benefits and joys of that experience. And there are also many labyrinthine structures, for example in the ways that plants grow, or in the shape of the small intestine or the circulatory system, the internal structure of the ear, or the winding streets of many cities and towns. The logic of the labyrinth is the logic of the fractal geometry, including the Peano curve, aka the space-filling curve. The pattern also applies to the oral tradition, its multiformity, variability, and homeostatic qualities, which Matthews explains is very much characteristic of the myths surrounding the Minotaur, Theseus, and Ariadne. As a structure that straddles the distinction between the linear and the nonlinear, the labyrinth also informs the path that *Ariadne Then and Now* follows, a winding stroll through mind and memory, wandering but never, ever lost.

More than anything else, the labyrinth is the metaphor and metapattern for life, for the kind of journey characteristic of human life. Not a straight line from beginning to middle to end, but a wandering along mysterious pathways, never knowing quite where we are or when we will arrive at our destination, or what awaits us along the way. As a memoir, and especially as the third edition of a memoir, Carol Matthews provides a profound reflection on life, and especially on end of life. Death is a subject that we go to great lengths to avoid in contemporary western culture, and yet it is an eventuality that we all must face, for ourselves, for those close to our hearts, and for the strangers in our midst and in our media environment who we become connected to, and who we encounter with empathy. The denial of death that so dominates contemporary life leaves us lost in the labyrinth, whereas the only way out, as Corey Anton makes clear, is through death acceptance. Carol Matthews shows great courage in *Ariadne Then and Now*, in facing her Minotaur, and coming to terms with the beast. In doing so, she reminds us that the interconnectedness of the social and biological worlds are labyrinths too, and that the thread that we need to follow, to set ourselves free, is that of ecology, of ecological thinking, of relations and relationships.

Simply put, *Ariadne Then and Now*, is a journey well worth taking, one that can help us along and help us get along, as we travel along the meandering routes, crisscrossing pathways, and spiraling circuits that we encounter in the living of our lives.

Lance Strate
Fordham University

A Guide to the Labyrinth

Some people use the labyrinth as a reflective practice that helps them to solve problems. Some use it as a way of dealing with illness, grief and loss. Some find it a calming, walking meditation, or a way of pursuingcreativity. For some, labyrinths and mazes simply provide an attractivefocus in a garden landscape, or a place of peaceful contemplation.

The winding path has deep roots spiraling back to early cave drawings, ancient buildings in Northern Egypt, Rome and Greece. For 4,000 years or more, labyrinths have appeared in countries around the world—in Scandinavia, Russia, Arizona and Peru. Labyrinth historian Jeff Saward tells us that the earliest labyrinth for which a precise date has been established is on a Linear B inscribed clay tablet from southern Greece in 1200 BCE. However, although it is difficult to date the earliest labyrinths, Saward notes that some of the carvings on rockfaces in Galicia, Spain are likely to have been created between 2500 to 1800 BC.

There are many types of labyrinths. They may be round, square, octagonal or of an irregular shape. The two designs most commonly seen are the "Cretan" or "Classical" labyrinth and the "Medieval" or"Chartres-style" labyrinth.

The Classical labyrinth is an early pattern which was associated with the labyrinth at Knossos, Greece and the mythological Minotaurwho was housed at its centre. The Medieval labyrinth is a more complex pattern which was adopted by the early Christian churchesand cathedrals, most famously at the Chartres cathedral near Paris.

There are also Native American designs such as the Man-in-the-Maze which offer a variation on the circular theme as well as some new forms such as the Santa Rosa Labyrinth, created by Dr. LeaGoode-Harris, and the Chalice labyrinth designed by Robert Peach.

The labyrinth may be seen as a metaphor for life's journey, but the Cretan myth of the Minotaur tells the story of a journey towardsdeath. Today as I walk the labyrinth I am thinking about the end of times. When I was undergoing treatment for breast cancer two years ago, walking this labyrinth grounded me to better face the unknowns of that situation. These days I walk the labyrinth because I have a sense that it will help me to reflect on much larger questions: what is the shape and meaning of my life? how can I learn to accept the realities of old age and approaching death? This quiet eleven-circuit Medieval labyrinth is surrounded by trees and flowers and offers a tranquil setting for such reflection and speculation.

The labyrinth is a winding path, and so my own story meanders slowly, moving towards and retreating from the centre. Anyone eager to get to the heart of things will not have the patience to accompany me on this journey for I will coil in and out, back and forth, like an elderly serpent. I do not expect that I will, when I reach the centre, shed this wrinkled old skin and emerge newborn, but some change will occur. I feel sure of that.

And, although it is a self-directed journey, I want someone to guide me. Charlotte, my six-year-old granddaughter, recently gave me advice she referred to as "two deep, dark secrets."

"It's a good idea to think of people who lived a very long time ago," she said.

And "It's a good idea to close your eyes when you really want to think about something."

I have no idea what she was talking about, but the instructions seem harmless, and so, standing with my eyes closed in the centre of this labyrinth, I think of someone who lived a very long time ago—Ariadne, the Mistress of the ancient Labyrinth in Knossos. I conjure her up.

Years ago, I saw a print of Waterhouse's Ariadne, titian-haired, flowing red robes, abandoned by Theseus, eyes closed in a deep swoon, but the image that comes to me now is of a tall, slender woman with shoulder length blond hair and eyes the blue-green shade of an Ionian sea. She wears a white Grecian tunic and her unbound hair ripples like waves as she walks toward me. She has the light step of a young girl, yet her body radiates the appetite and desire of a more mature woman

I present her with a question: To die and face not being—how to do it? More important, how to move through these last years, 'the end zone,' with a fine finish?

2

Think of your origins. You must look back to see ahead.

Walking back and forth on this stone and turf labyrinth, following the inescapable, one-way path, I look back and speculate on thechoices I made in my life, the many roads not taken. I wonder what those alternate endings might have been for me. Might they have been better ones?

You're looking for the happy ending? Her voice is flute-like, lyrical, with a hint of an ancient accent. *In our time, we thought not of such things.*

It's not just about happy ending. It's about alternate endings. Anyway, there were never any happy endings in your myths.

Myths?

Stories, then. Histories. Like the Minotaur in your labyrinth.

Ah yes. My half-brother. Asterion. His story was not a happy one. Poseidon caused my mother, Passiphae, to become infatuated with a bull in order to punish the greed of my father, King Minos. My mother copulated with the white bull, and from that union came the Minotaur.

It's hard to imagine how your mother could actually have had sex with a bull.

It wasn't easy. My mother summoned Daedalus, the great inventor, to create a decoy she could use in order to attract the bull and satisfy her passion. Daedalus built her a hollow wooden cow covered with a cow's hide—a cow suit—and he showed her how to slip inside and thrust her legs into the cow's hindquarters.

Ingenious! And yet...

Daedalus was clever. Within the structure, he built a small trap door so that the bull could actually mount Passiphae. And that's how my half-brother was conceived. Born with a human body and a bull's head, he was known as the Minotaur and condemned to live his life as a monster until eventually he was slain by Theseus.

It's puzzling. The ancient Greeks had many hybrid creatures in their midst. There were centaurs, creatures with the head of a man and the body of a horse. There were satyrs with goat-like features. There were harpies and Gorgons, female monsters with snake hair,fangs, claws and wings. People were always copulating with animals. They enjoyed it.

Why was your brother seen to be such a problem, given all the other half-humans?

Half-brother. He needn't have been a problem. You must understand that the real story about our labyrinth had little to do with Asterion, much to do with the machinations of men. My father, King Minos of Crete, and Theseus's father, King Aegeus of Athens, never got along. There were old rivalries and resentments, as with your own rulers. When my father had Daedalus build a labyrinth to house the Minotaur, he also ordered that every ninth year the Athenians should send seven youths and seven maidens to be devoured by him.

In short, your father used the Minotaur as a weapon to punish King Aegeus. And it took Theseus to put an end to it?

Yes. Every ninth year the youths and maidens arrived. Or perhaps every third year. There are different versions of the story. Each time they were overcome by Asterion. It had always been my job to prepare them for the massacre, and I didn't enjoy it at all. It was a bloody business, and in the end, I was relieved when Theseus came to slay Asterion. Eventually I would have had to do it myself.

Why did they keep coming?

I did wonder about that.

The peaceful setting of the retreat centre here is in sharp contrast to the grisly place that Ariadne describes. I'm lucky I didn't live in that time.

Count no one lucky until she is dead, my friend. Life is a labyrinth, and it is not for the faint of heart.

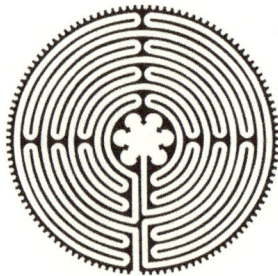

Returning to Labyrinths, Aging and Death

I'm winding my way around a stone path, thinking about the monster at its centre and asking questions of Ariadne. Why did you need Theseus to help in dealing with the Minotaur? You knew your way around those twists and turns.

Theseus was an attractive man and he liked being a hero. In any case, Asterion was my half-brother. My job was to care for him, not to slaughter him.

Asterion?

Star. Named after my maternal grandfather, another Asterion. The men in my family were always stars.

In my own family the men were also stars, while women were—what? The Milky Way? A diffuse image of nurturing? Insignificant bodies destined to disappear into black holes? The pattern is a familiar one.

My brothers were brought up to do something in the world. They were the meteors, the real stars. I was just supposed to be a nice girl and stay out of trouble. Not a really demanding task, but I quit it early, though not to become a star. Quitting was my custom.

Nonetheless, you have arrived at this advanced age...

And now I'm reflecting on my origins, Ariadne. Just as you advised.

Origins can be convoluted. Nothing starts at the beginning. There's always the story before the story. My father was also conceived from a trick with a bull. His father, Zeus, disguised himself as a bull in order to seduce my grandmother, Europa. The difference is that my grandmother's bull had an excellent pedigree so my father, unlike Asterion, was not born with the physical features of a monster.

My own lineage appears more straightforward, yet as soon as I think this, I realize that there are many mysteries in my own family history. Like Zeus and Europa, my parents had little in common when they met. Their families of origin, from different social classes, his from the North of England, hers from the South,

5

could not have been more dissimilar. My grandparents would have thought such a match inconceivable. An inter-species union.

There are also the stories beside the story. The alternate paths. The might-have-beens.

I have no way of figuring all that out. Trying to recover those pasts and those paths is like trying to piece together a puzzle in which there are blank spaces on all sides. What I want to know is how I got to this place and how I can carry on to the next one. Life is not for the faint of heart, you say. I will need to strengthen my heart so that I can face the end of times.

Be patient, my friend. The labyrinth is not a maze. Follow the path inwards and then outwards, from side to side. It will help you to understand where you have been and where you are going.

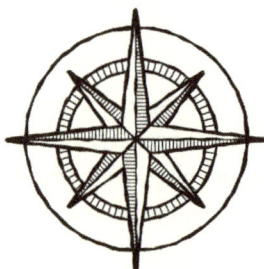

Labyrinths and Mazes

"Why don't they make these labyrinths more vertical?" my husband asks, as we walk together on a handsome outdoor labyrinth born of stone and gravel. This eleven-circuit Chartres-style labyrinth is wonderfully situated in a quiet, forested area where one hears the stream running along beside the glade. "It would be more mysterious if there were high hedges."

"You're thinking of mazes. Hampton Court in England, or the Giardino Giusti in Verona. They both have high hedges. That's how you get lost. But that's not the purpose of a labyrinth."

"I know that you can't get lost in a labyrinth, but I think it would be a more interesting experience if it were three-dimensional."

"You're supposed to be able to see the pattern and you can't do that with a maze. And in the labyrinth, you get to see the other walkers so you have the sense of being part of a larger group."

Mike looks skeptical. He'd rather walk alone

The Oxford English Dictionary defines "labyrinth" and "maze" as synonyms. My *Women's Dictionary of Symbols & Sacred Objects* distinguishes a labyrinth as having only one path, "winding but branchless, heading inevitably toward the goal," and claims the design was first scratched or carved on Stone Age monuments and grave sites to represent the soul's journey into the center of the underworld and its return, reborn.

While the labyrinth and the maze are both spiritual symbols, beautiful and significant, they are now usually defined as two very different patterns, each with its distinct purpose and outcome. The labyrinth is a simple, straightforward path, while the maze is a complex and confusing one. Trust and intuition guide the labyrinth walker; strategy and deduction are required in the maze. The labyrinth can be used as a tool for contemplation and reflection; the maze is a puzzle to be solved, designed to trick the walker. The labyrinth has a unicursal path—the way in is also the way out— while the maze is multicursal, with many possible directions and lots of blind alleys. Sometimes, in our life and work, we seem to be in a labyrinth and then, all of a sudden, we find ourselves up against a wall, faced with dead ends, immersed in a maze, with no apparent way out. You need strategy to find your way out of a maze.

H.D. Kitto, a renowned scholar on Greek civilization, tells us that the Cretans worshipped the bull and that the ground plan of the palace in Knossos that British archaeologist Arthur Evans dug up looks like a labyrinth. He recounts the story of Theseus slaying the monster in the labyrinth at Knossos, and says it is clear that the Cretans worshipped the bull. Much of the story is true. But nobody, he says, has substantiated "the romantic Ariadne" or found the legendary string, the golden thread that she gave to Theseus. I wonder just what Ariadne thinks about all this.

My father employed Daedalus to build the original labyrinth at Knossos. It was a trap designed to contain the Minotaur, and it did so for many years. That's how it was, how it all began.

I don't understand how the classical labyrinth could have contained the Minotaur. The maze might work as a trap, but not the labyrinth.

The Minotaur could not escape.

But other people must have found their way in and out. They had to feed the Minotaur. And clean out his quarters.

That was my job. I knew the labyrinth inside and out. But most of the people who entered did not return.

The Minotaur devoured them, year after year.

Every few years. Some say every nine years, some say three. I didn't keep track. There are so many different stories about the labyrinth. Amazing stories.

I don't believe people ever spoke of mazes in your time, did they?

Nor did we speak much about the labyrinth. It was just what it was. A simple pattern. Inasmuch as any spiral can be called simple.

Spirals. I wonder just how much Ariadne knows of this ancient pattern. The spirals scratched or carved on monuments, caves and grave sites, long before Ariadne's time. Those early drawings of bulls' heads and horns are seen by scholars such as Maria Gimbutas to symbolize the uterus and fallopian tubes, representing the female power of generativity.

Is it possible that the real story about the labyrinth is not about Theseus, not the hero's but the heroine's journey? After all, it was she who was in charge of the Labyrinth. And it was she who consulted Daedalus the labyrinth builder, then offered the sage advice and golden thread to Theseus. Did Ariadne, like so many of us, choose to be an enabler instead of an actor?

Why didn't you slay the Minotaur, Ariadne? You knew how to escape the labyrinth.

Asterion and I are of one flesh. I had to care for him. And Theseus was training to be a hero. He needed the opportunity.

Weren't you disappointed when Theseus, having successfully defeated the Minotaur and made his escape, abandoned you on the island of Naxos?

Yes, but in the end, it was for the best. Aphrodite took pity on me and told me that I would have an immortal lover. That's when Dionysus came along, Naxos being one of his favourite islands. He fell in love with me instantly and lifted me to live with him among the gods on Mount Olympus.

So, you went from the labyrinth at Knossos to what must have at first appeared to be a perplexing maze on Naxos and then, with a sudden turn of events, the journey led you to an entirely new path as an immortal goddess, wife of Dionysus?

Press on with your explorations, my friend. Find the Minotaur at the centre of your own labyrinth.

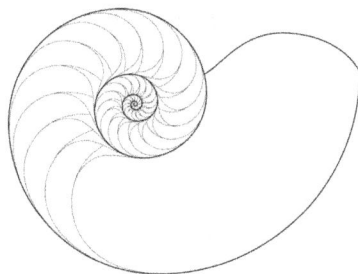

Deep Down

What is it in the labyrinth that has so captured my imagination? The circles, for a start. Years ago, studying symbolic logic, I was only ever able to find the solutions by a circuitous route. The professor said he could never see where I was going. He was impressed when I came up with the right answer, but declared that a shorter, direct route was "more elegant." I've always fancied the longer, curved path. The winding labyrinth is a fitting instrument for my quest.

I concentrate on my physical being. The circles calm and center me, giving me a sense that the labyrinth will provide shape to my life. At the same time, as I walk step by step on the varnished floor, I think it might be a slippery slope down to the invisible, death-dealing beast at the centre. I am approaching my own personal Minotaur.

Lots of people have been fascinated by the Minotaur—Borges. Jung. Picasso. In New York, some years ago, at the Museum of Modern Art, I saw Picasso's *Le Minotauromachy*, a painting in which an enormous bull-headed Minotaur confronts a young girl who holds a candle and a bouquet of flowers. A wounded female matador rides a rearing horse, and sacrificial girls hold doves. The same horrific images as in Guernica, his famous anti-war mural about the horrorsof Fascism. *Le Minotauromachy* is also seen as reflecting the turmoil in Picasso's own life, his personal demons at a time when his marriage was troubled and his mistress pregnant. Because I am writing about death, the dark path to the Minotaur takes on a personal shape for me as well.

As a child, I frequently awakened to nightmares of ghostly figures in murky tunnels. My first grade was at a one-room school in what was then a rural area, a setting which still holds dark corners in my imagination. The teacher was a wispy, woodsy creature who seemed, mysteriously, to emerge from the forest each morning. She taught us how to make 'marbled' designs by swirling pigments in a tray of water and laying paper on top to pick up the intricate winding patterns, and she wrote scripts for theatrical performances, in one of which I wore a Grecian tunic and stood by an imaginary window saying, "Oh dear, what a dull day!" After that performance we went downstairs into the basement to take off our costumes, and suddenly the janitor, an enormous, bearded man, burst in, ordered us all outside, and loudly demanded if someone had tinkered with the plumbing. When I ventured that I had touched one of the faucets, he strode over, bent down close to my face, and shouted, "You are a stupid little girl, aren't you?" Whether or not I caused the flooded basement, I will never forget the sense of being responsible for the deluge.

Now, many decades later, when my granddaughter, Charlotte, comes to stay, I sometimes awaken to her cries in the night and her explanation that there were 'bad guys' in her dream. When I ask her to tell me about the nightmare she says, no, she doesn't want to speak about it. Already she senses that when fears are given words,they gain substance.

Ted Hughes was fascinated by the bull-headed man. In his poem "The Minotaur" he writes about the need to confront the damage that the Minotaur can do, about "the bloody end of the skein" that left children "echoing like tunnels in a labyrinth." The monster, the bloody skein, the tunnels of the labyrinth—these are the stuff of nightmares, always lurking in the netherworld. Here is the shadow world that contains those things that we don't know or don't want to know. "Everyone carries a shadow," Jung says, "and the less it is embodied in the individual's conscious life, the blacker and denser it is."

It's been several years since my cancer diagnosis, but the shadowy fears do not lessen. Fears about something malignant within me, hidden from sight. I feel like one of those early cartographers who inscribed uncharted regions with the words *Hic sunt dracones*, sometimes decorating their maps with drawings of the fearsome dragon creatures rising from the water or devouring wayward ships. Dark things, rising up from the deep.

I need to continue, to follow Ariadne into the core of the labyrinth, face the darkness and find my innermost self, but I hesitate, backing away from such explorations. I remember visiting Douglas Hospital, the old mental institution in Montreal with its dank, underground corridors. That, I think, is where a journey of self-discovery might take me. Backwards into the murky tunnels of my youth. Onwards to the labyrinth of life and death.

Especially death. The Cretan labyrinth, with its story of Ariadne, Theseus, and the Minotaur, may have been created as a map to theUnderworld, leading the departing souls down into the afterlife. In Arizona, the Man in the Maze pattern is said to represent the long, winding upward path leading to the home of the Navajo ancestors. Upward or downward, I'm captivated by the winding pattern.

Our bodies contain spirals, and they too can harbour monsters,as in the case of my friend Rose, whose cancer causes blockage of the bowel, that inner human labyrinth. Brains too resemble labyrinths. I recently watched a video that has been circulating over the internet,one of the TED talks in which a brain scientist spoke of waking up one morning to realize she was having a stroke. She tells the story of her experience and shows images of how our neural circuitry operates. Watching the video, I couldn't help but notice the labyrinthine look of the neurological images, the cerebral spirals.

Fibonacci spiraling sequences are in daisies and roses and pinecones. In the dazzling clockwise and counterclockwise seed patterns of sunflowers. In snail shells, vines, galaxies. Spirals are in our brains, bowels,and inner ears. In the double helix of our DNA. And the spiral is also the central seed of the labyrinths and mazes which have wound their circuitous paths on rockfaces, courtyards, cathedral floors, and gardens and beaches all around our planet.

When I walk the circuitous roads of the tiny island on which I live, I have the sense that it too is a kind of labyrinth. Or perhaps a maze. No road is straight. All curve, and wind, and interconnect.

More and more, wherever I look, I see myriad spiraling, labyrinthine connections. Coincidences and convergences, out of which I can make no sense whatsoever.

For the moment, contemplating old age and death, it is Ariadne's winding thread I choose to follow.

Come, my friend. It's normal to be afraid of the unknown, especially as you approach the monstrosities of illness and old age. But the journey must be taken. The connections must be made.

The Minotaur in the Garden

My husband has become quite interested in labyrinths, despite his initial skepticism.

"The walking is a helpful reflective practice," I explain. "It calms me. And the labyrinth myth, the story of the Minotaur is a meaningful one that can give shape to your life."

"I don't like these woo woo activities," he used to say, "these practices. Why don't people just stay home and read *The Greeks*, by Kitto, as I did?"

But now the winding paths are drawing him in to a meditative journey, whether he likes it or not, so he's receptive to my proposal to take Charlotte to see an outdoor labyrinth in a botanical garden.

"It's called a Cretan labyrinth," I tell Charlotte, "and it's unusual because there is an actual Minotaur there."

"That's strange," she says, "and it's also odd. I didn't think real labyrinths had Minotaurs anymore." For a six-year-old, she knows quite a lot about labyrinths and has walked a number of them with me. We've also done some tracing of labyrinths and mazes on paper, and I've told her the story of Ariadne's labyrinth at Knossos, omitting some of the gruesome details.

"But you like strange and odd things, don't you?"

Charlotte gives me a piercing glance and says, "I don't like it when they kill the bull. I don't think people should kill animals."

"Well, this wasn't a regular animal. He was a monster, half-human and half-beast."

"I still don't like it. And I don't like the word 'beast.'"

Arriving at the gardens, we are met by deep red rhododendrons, brilliant azaleas, creamy and crimson magnolias, the ancient gingko, towering hemlocks, and enormous Douglas firs. Charlotte races ahead through the looping woodland walks, exclaiming over the flowering shrubs, disappearing and reappearing every few minutes. Mike and I explore along with her, trying to discover where a labyrinth might be hidden in all this abundance.

Every search for these mysterious structures takes us on circuitous routes, but eventually we locate the tunnel that leads to the

Cretan labyrinth. Here, at the beginning of the seven-circuit pathway, is a Minotaur, designed by British artist Sophie Ryder. Seven feet tall, he's constructed of a wire frame and covered with swirls and whorls of twigs and vines. A real woodland creature. In his paws he holds a small blue hare, cupping it tenderly in just the way, it seems to me, that my husband might hold a cheeseburger or a bacon and tomato sandwich. "What's the Minotaur going to do with that rabbit?" Charlotte asks with an expression of deep distrust.

"Maybe they're just making friends with each other." I propose that the artist might want to draw those two mismatched creatures together into a state of harmony. I've seen photographs of other works in which she brings a hare together with various animals and demonstrates their potential for affection. This sculpture suggests the possibility of co-existence, and nicely subverts the Theseus story to propose options for the Minotaur.

"They're making friends?" Charlotte asks. "Why not?"

That settles it. Charlotte announces that she'll lead the way and starts out on the path. This turf labyrinth is soft and yielding underfoot, but I call out a warning because the Canadian geese who are wandering nearby have left a heavy offering of turds in their wake.

I like the easy flow to this path. It's a gentler, faster walk than the Chartres-style labyrinth, with a greater feeling of openness and accessibility. Certainly this labyrinth, with its evident entry and exit, could never actually contain any kind of creature. Anyone could make an easy escape, which is perhaps why Ryder's Minotaur is just outside the entrance. He's on the loose!

I stay in the labyrinth to commune with Ariadne while Charlotte and Mike go over to examine the Minotaur.

"I'm glad he isn't in a prison. I like him, and so does the rabbit." I hear Charlotte announce.

She has an Olympian spirit. Perhaps she can show you the way.

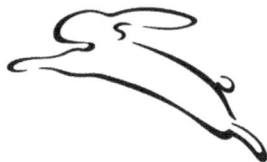

Facing Death

There is something delightful about a labyrinth that is constructed of turf and wildflowers, surrounded by evergreens on one side and bordered with brilliant swaths of lavender on the other. Inside this labyrinth are tiny white daisies, yellow buttercups and purple clover, and the ground here is accommodating, full of mystery. Close to the centre is a stone bench on which to sit while looking out at either the tall cedars, or the rows of lavender with their various shades of blue and purple. Beside the bench is a stone circled by a variety of thyme. The woman who designed this labyrinth speaks of the many gifts people of diverse faiths gave when the labyrinth was opened. A man who holds Wicca beliefs brought a tablet inscribed with symbols and placed it under the centre stone. Not visible, it suggests the way things are always hidden in the labyrinth, the many layers of meaning that one encounters. I think it would be nice to be, like that tablet, buried here, another hidden, underground presence.

What did the Greeks think of burial? I envision Ariadne, seated at the centre of the labyrinth, weaving daisy and lavender into a wreath.

We believed that people died only on the ebb tide. Of course, lots of cultures believed that. In with the high, out with the low.

Were people buried at sea?

Hermes would lead the dead souls down to the River Styx which divides the living world from the other world. Charon would ferry the dead souls across the river to the underworld.

And then you were left to live among the dead?

The underworld had its own population, all the shadowy people who have died. The shades, Hades and Persephone, reigned in that territory deep down under the earth. It was just another state of being, but not a really happy place.

It sounds scary.

Not as scary as the space in between the worlds. The liminal space, which is not really a place at all, merely a flux between this world and the beyond.

That's where I am now, Ariadne. Old age is the liminal space. You don't know when it happened, but suddenly there is a transition into unfamiliar territory and you realize that you lack the knowledge and skills to find your way.

You are still alive, my friend. Concentrate on living well.

Ariadne stands up and places her white and purple flowered wreath on her head. Lovely and ageless, she is a symbol of the life on Mount Olympus.

Easy for her to be optimistic, but how are we non-Olympians to face the final years? That's the question I want answered. I've decided that over the next six months I will reflect on the seven tasks that Jung set out for successful aging:

Task No. 1: Facing the Reality of Aging and Dying
Task No. 2: Conducting a Life Review
Task No. 3: Defining Life Realistically
Task No. 4: Letting Go of the Ego
Task No. 5: Finding a New Rooting in the Self
Task No. 6: Determining the Meaning of One's Life
Task No. 7: Rebirth—Dying with Life.

Task No. 7 seems to be a deathbed operation and the first task is unavoidable, but I'll see how far I can get with the remaining five. I find a website that lists 45 signs of aging. "Not an exhaustive list," it says, but I don't intend to read them.

Not everyone agrees that aging needs to be faced. Recently I was talking to a friend who told me she was going to write a book called "Aging is not an Option." When I rolled my eyes, she insisted, "Really, it's just *not* an option these days. You have to do whatever it takes to stay young." She's about fifteen years my junior and looks at least fifteen years younger than her actual age. She looks after herself and is careful about fitness, hair colour, make-up, dress. It's a considerable time investment, but one she considers necessary.

There are some women who see aging as providing new and attractive options. In an article in *The Guardian*, Alison Lurie wrote about realizing that, after reaching 60, she didn't have to pursue fashion anymore but could wear the old clothes she loved and comfortable shoes, that she could stop colouring her hair and could throw away her make-up. She describes a joyful sense of self-determination that accompanies freedom from the prescriptions of fashionable magazines, a freedom which offers greater ease and also saves a good deal of time. The freedom we had as children.

I'm ready to face the reality of aging but I have yet to find comfort in the fact. Some would claim that age brings wisdom and clarity, as in "Land of the Blind," 17th century Edmund Waller's verse on old age:

> *The soul's dark cottage, batter'd and decay'd,*
> *Lets in new light through chinks that Time hath made:*
> *Stronger by weakness, wiser men become*
> *As they draw near to their eternal home.*

Mike objects to that word "cottage," says it is too much like a greeting card, but I find the notion of new light being let in through "chinks" made by time to be comforting.

"The idea of death doesn't bother me," Mike announces, "Like Woody Allen, I just don't want to be there when it happens." His approach to anything unpleasant is simple avoidance and denial.

"It's not that I'm afraid of death," I tell him. "I don't even mind being there when it happens. It's the possibility of being incapacitated that terrifies me. I don't want to end my life in a nursing home."

This is the fear which haunts us all. We've seen parents and older friends restricted to wheelchairs, eking out days and nights in geriatric institutions, their last sad days and months and years overshadowing the brighter times of their early lives. And the last days lengthen as our life expectancy increases. I read somewhere that for every day you live your life expectancy goes up another five hours. Curious as it seems, the longer you live, the longer you can expect to live. But for how long in good health? The reality of aging is that it often brings disability, dependency, dementia. I've read reports that suggest you can expect to live at least ten years longer than your healthy life expectancy projection. How to prepare for that? Facing death is one thing, the realities of advanced old age is quite another. Our projected death edges further away, hour by hour, day by day, while the years of incapacity loom longer and increasingly inescapable. Surely we should spend the intervening years fighting for assisted suicide.

My father as a robust middle-aged man used to recite or sing "Invictus," delivering those brave lines in his hearty bass voice:

> Beyond this place of wrath and tears
> Looms but the Horror of the shade
> And yet the menace of the years
> Finds, and shall find, me unafraid.

For the most part, he maintained this spirit, never whimpering under "bludgeonings of age and disability." When in his later years Parkinson's Disease left him unable to speak, let alone sing, I was often reminded of the lyrics of another of his other favourite songs, *Old Man River*. Of Paul Robeson singing "Ah'm tired of livin'/An' skeered of dyin'." A sentiment shared by many.

It's baffling to me that Carl Jung called the first task for successful aging "Facing the Reality of Aging and Dying." How can you possibly avoid facing the reality of aging when every day it's literallyin your face—and on your face—whenever you look in the mirror? The brown spots that suddenly appear on the face and hands. The seborrheic keratoses, odd little growths that some call "the barnaclesof old age." Forgetfulness, poor night vision, bad knees, loss of hearing, interrupted sleep.

The signs start gradually and then quickly creep up on you so that the real awareness that one is becoming old and things are drawing to a close always comes as a shock. We get in the habit of looking ahead as though our time could be endless, and then suddenly here we are, in a different place, facing a future that may be very different from the one we'd planned. At the center of the labyrinth I often contemplate exactly this question: should I stay right on to the end, even if it is not what I intended?

When I consider the options, I'm drawn to the solution of "the long swim," a simple, elegant and final strategy by which you swim out a distance, well beyond the returning point, figuring in the tidesand currents, and choose the precise moment at which there will beno possibility of return. Timing is everything. I frequently propose it to my husband. He declines, despite the fact that he detests old age even more than I do.

18

"Old age! Impossible, humiliating," Mike says, "not to be endured!" And yet it is not really so bad for men. Unlike women, I point out, men may be attractive even when quite old. In fact, although now in his seventies, my husband is still handsome. I tell him so, and he says, "I'm all right now, but what about when I have little white arms, hanging over my flabby paunch?" I assure him that I have met very old men who are captivating. Charming. "Not when they have little white arms," he says.

He doesn't like the idea of advanced old age, nor does he like the idea of suicide. Or euthanasia. Or rather, he likes it in principle, but not as it might apply to him in the foreseeable future. I, however, think we should try to find ways of helping to ease suffering at the end of life. I will wish this for myself one day, so I would like to work to make it available.

Otherwise, there's only the prospect of the two of us wading out together. Bathing suits all wrinkled, like second skins covering our own loose white flesh. Our sensitive old feet shod in new beach shoes to protect them from the sharp rocks. Our flaccid limbs, pale and mottled, diminished. The icy waters would lap at our feet and my husband would reach out, when I hesitated at the water's edge. He would wrap one tiny little white arm around my shoulder and lead me slowly into the dark blue waves, the deepening waters. But whenever my imagination reaches this point I see him turn and swim strongly back to the shore as I flounder in the depths.

Find your own direction, my friend. The choice is yours.

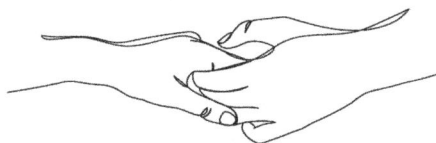

The Dark and the Light

I've come to Toronto to see my friend Rose. She told the hospital staff that she doesn't want extraordinary measures, and so now they've told her that she should arrange to see the people she wants to see, say the things that need to be said. So, she's asked me to come.

Before going to the hospital, I stop at the downtown labyrinth that was developed by the Labyrinth Community Network in collaboration with the City of Toronto and The Church of the Holy Trinity. This labyrinth is a handsome stone construction nestled beside a hundred and sixty-year-old church that offers services in English and Spanish. Surrounded by skyscrapers in the midst of the concrete jungle of downtown Toronto, the labyrinth is surprisingly empty. Don't all those people in those rabbit warrens that constitute their workplacesfeel the need to clear their heads sometimes? This lovely path should be chock-full of meditators!

As I enter the labyrinth, my thoughts are about Rose, about illness, about the fear of death. Like me, Rose was diagnosed with cancer two years ago, but hers is a more dire type, and the disease has progressed rapidly. So many of my friends are growing old, becoming ill. In my mind, a brain worm of that old hymn, *Abide with Me*, twists around. *Change and decay in all around I see...On to the close, O Lord, abide with me*. The man who wrote that hymn was Reverend Henry Lyte, pastor at a poor parish church at Lower Brixham in Devonshirewho, just weeks before his death, wrote those lyrics about change and decay and the fading of the light. It's said that on the day of hislast sermon, in 1847, he was so ill he practically had to crawl to the pulpit to tell his parishioners to prepare for the solemn hour.

Rose squarely faces the severity of her condition, knows that final hour is approaching, yet she does not seem to be preparing for death. On the contrary, she is full of vitality.

"Rose is like the sun," I used to say. "As soon as she enters a room, you feel the warmth of her presence, and everything around her brightens up. But if you get too close to the sun, you can get burnt." Even when we spoke on the telephone a few days ago, thousands of miles apart, I could feel Rose's extraordinary power, although it's dwindling now. Until recently she entertained lavishly, her style commanding attention and respect, but it's not like the days when she lived with Pierre. The amazing old days. Those two were like Beatrice and Benedick, Zelda and Scott, Eloise and Abelard, Antony and Cleopatra—all the great lovers you have ever known rolled into one. Even their names made them seem like some kind of fairy tale couple. The Rose and the Rock. She once told me about a game the two of them played together, a variation on Jan-Ken-Pon, that Japanese hand game. Only their version was Rose-Rock-Spear and it was played in bed.

That's how I think of Rose. As she was in those days, before Pierre died, before she became ill. Now, as I walk the labyrinth's winding path, I feel Rose is helping me to ready myself to meet theMinotaur, that deathly spectre at the centre.

Olympians don't ever really die. We just disappear for awhile.

Yet death is everywhere in your stories.

Death is everywhere, but we ourselves just sort of fade away, and then after awhile we reappear. As though to prove her point, she disappears.

Being an Olympian has definite advantages, yet I feel a bit sorry for Ariadne. Her life has not been without challenges. First that grislyjob, watching all the youths and maidens get slaughtered every how-ever many years. Then doing all that work for Theseus—getting him the golden thread, waiting at the gate of the labyrinth, drugging the guards, releasing other prisoners, setting off to Naxos—only to windup abandoned on a small island.

I keep wondering how it might have gone if she'd faced the monster herself. She was smart enough to consult Daedalus, yet rather than going in and becoming the hero, she gave the silken thread—the "golden clew"—and the good advice to Theseus.

And look where that led you. I summon Ariadne back. Weren't you furious?

Of course. And I was heartbroken. But Theseus was like that. An excitable boy. Forgetful. He forgot all about me, and he also failed to remember that he should hoist the white sails to signal his victory. Aegeus,his father, seeing the black sails, believed that Theseus must be dead and flung himself from a cliff.

21

From what I've read in Greek mythology, your people seem to have had a habit of flinging yourselves or others from cliffs!

It was preferable to a lingering death. In any case, Theseus promptly forgot about all that, and went on to abduct a few other women, my sister Phaedra among them. He married her.

Your sister agreed to marry him, after the way he'd treated you?

Before or after, depending upon who is telling the story. Phaedra was another victim of the family pathology. You may have read about how she fell in love with her stepson, Theseus's son, Hippolytus.

Your nephew?

I have a large family. Phaedra's story was an unhappy one, in every version that is told. Some say Aphrodite caused Phaedra to develop that incestuous passion out of jealousy, but I doubt it. Aphrodite was always good to me. However, my sister suffered great grief and eventually she committed suicide.

Another cliff?

No. Euripides claims she died of poison, but I believe she hanged herself. It's always been something of a mystery. But then every death is its own mystery.

A clutch of children arrives at the labyrinth and begins a wild race to see which of them can first reach the centre and, then, who can first find the way out. I expect they might have preferred a maze to a labyrinth, but they're having fun and it's consoling to hear their laughter. No thoughts of the Minotaur, Sybils, death rituals, or the underworld haunt their journey. Nor any thought of endings, happy or otherwise.

At the Princess Margaret Hospital, a group of Rose's friends collect in the waiting room. People gather around the dying the way crows collect to circle a wounded bird—helpless to heal but watching, waiting. I know that more of such moments are ahead for me, just out of sight, just around a corner. The recognition of impending death. It makes me quiver to think it. My mother would say, "Someone just walked over my grave." She'd been told by her grandmother that, although we don't know where we will be buried, something in us trembles when our future grave is walked upon. Just an old superstition, my mother assured me, yet it was what she always said when something made her shudder.

Despite her age and illness, Rose retains her amazing good looks and wants all the things around her to be the very best they can be. Books are stacked neatly, photographs are carefully placed, and the dozens of cards are not on display but tidily tucked away for future reference. On the bedside tray are expensive lotions, a Chanel lipstick and a pretty silver mirror engraved with her initials. A blown glass vase brought from home sits on the windowsill. The pale white peonies it holds are made from paper because patients are not per- mitted fresh flowers in their rooms. The reason for this, I am told, is that there may be bacteria on plants and flowers. All the plants and flowers sent to patients are collected at the nursing station, but surely the risks can only be concentrated and intensified by this ac- cumulation. I fear for the health of the nurses!

It's hard to believe Rose can actually be dying. She doesn't look so very different, yet the disease progresses unseen in her bowels. It is as Blake described so well:

O Rose, thou art sick
The invisible worm,
That flies in the night
In the howling storm:

Has found out thy bed
Of crimson joy:
And his dark secret love
Does thy life destroy.

Amidst the ambiguities, indignities, inefficiencies, discomforts and frustrations that are visited upon her, Rose is serene. It occurs to me that she's leading the way more than ever before, teaching me how to face the end of life, showing me the importance of making the best choices.

It's never too early to be conscious of how it will all end. I think of Robert Frost's poem, *Better to go down dignified...Provide. Provide.* But how should we provide? How can we finally detach?

Several times it has seemed to me that Rose was close to the end, and then she has rallied. She's on oxygen now, as well as intravenous and other tubes, yet she remains fully present, full of life, insisting on everything being the best it can be. I'm reminded of Anne Tyler's novel *Breathing Lessons*, at the end of which a man playing a chess game says that he'd come to the interesting part of the game where "the choices are fewer and every move counts."

Every move has always mattered to Rose, every single little thinghas counted. "Why can't things just be ordinary?" I used to ask her. "What's wrong with good enough?"

It would drive me crazy when she'd say, "No, no, let's walk on this side of the street, it's prettier," and, "We can't go to that restaurant because it's too ugly." Books must be brilliant, a holiday should be spent at the premiere resort on an incomparably beautiful Greek island. When I once told her about a builder's caution that putting in a skylight at the entrance of our house might create too much light, she scoffed, "Too much light! What would that look like?"

Your friend is a light-bearer like my husband's brother, Apollo. He was always going on about light and clarity.

Was your husband like that?

Dionysus was a wine-god. He liked to promote intoxication, disruption, enthusiasm and ecstasy.

Rose liked those things too.

A full life needs both. The dark and the light.

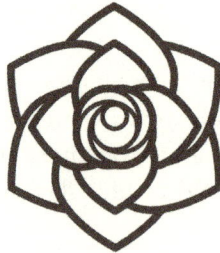

Reflections

Today I am at reading from my cancer memoir at an event organized by my publishers. On a pavement just outside the church is a Chartres-style labyrinth which was painted on the church parking lot by the rector several years earlier. Frequented by people of various ages, it welcomes all walkers, from the feeble elderly who pace it carefully to the lively children who race quickly through and around the path. I generally prefer the feeling of turf or sod underfoot to this unyielding pavement, but I do enjoy the peaceful sense created by the surrounding trees, with its view of the 123-year-old graveyard alongside the pretty church and the glimpses of the sea that lies just beyond.

Although the weather has been unseasonably cold, snow falling off and on throughout the day, it clears up enough that I am able to walk the labyrinth in comfort.

And what is your question today?

"It's a long story."

I have time. All the time in the world.

I tell her about the mirrored reflections I've seen of myself recently while examining the itchy spots that have appeared on my back. These spots feel bumpy and when I catch a glimpse of them in the mirror they look red and irritated. Not surprising, since I've been scratching at them.

At first I am reluctant to go to the doctor. This isn't the first time I've had bumps or rashes that concerned me, and mostly they've turned out to be "senile warts," which are merely irritating, benign symptoms of aging. I try to envision these changes as "transformations," putting a positive spin on deterioration. It's not easy.

My family doctor does not prescribe any treatment for the rash because, she says, she doesn't want it to get better.

"I don't mean I don't want it to get better *eventually*," she explains, laughing, "But I do want the dermatologist to see it just as it is now."

The dermatologist makes quick work of my symptoms, prescribing a cortisone cream to be applied thickly twice a day until the rash goes away. She has no explanation for the cause.

"They call it the *id reaction*," she explains, "because we just don't know why it happens." I suppose I look puzzled.

"Id," she repeats, "as in the unconscious. Freud."

I've been applying the medication she gave me, but I believe it should be possible to find other ways of alleviating my subterranean tensions. If I figure out what's troubling me, perhaps my skin will clear up. I recall the words of Joseph Campbell from a conference in Seattle long ago: "We cannot cure the world of its sorrows, but we can choose to live in joy." Good advice, but not so easy. For the moment I choose to pursue increasing my awareness of myself through the opportunities that the labyrinth offers for reflection.

One of the great reflectors of all times was Leonardo da Vinci. Most of what he wrote in his extensive notebooks was written backwards, so that it could only be read in reflection, when held up to a mirror. To keep his information secret? Because he was left-handed—writing from right to left in order not to smudge his pages? I prefer to think that he liked mystery and wanted to puzzle his readers, force them to reflect.

Leonardo was a brilliant man, but he didn't always conclude things. Only a few of his 17 paintings were actually finished to his satisfaction, and many other projects were left undone. For example, he envisioned and designed a bronze horse, but it was five hundred years later before that horse was actually built. He made plans for seashell-shaped churches, revolving bridges and flying machines that were never actually built. Most of his ideas were ahead of the time. He produced more than 3,500 pages of sketches and writings, including many drawings of labyrinths. Clearly, he wasn't a quitter like me, but rather an ambitious starter who was a visionary and a perfectionist.

I am particularly interested in one of his pen-and-ink drawings that Hermann Kern refers to in a compendium on labyrinths. Above the drawing, the word "mirror" is inscribed backwards in Italian. Below, also in reverse script, da Vinci proposes the construction of a mirrored octagon consisting of eight flat surfaces, 1.2 x 1.8 metres, so that "a man standing inside it can see himself infinitely from all sides." Unfortunately, this project couldn't be carried out because mirrors so large could not be made in Leonardo's time.

I wish someone would build it now. Imagine a labyrinth whose heart provides a 360-degree view of the person who enters it! A goodperspective from which to contemplate my *id reaction*, both the rash on my back and the inner landscape which underlies it.

Reflection is only the starting point. You must go further.

When I meet Ariadne's clear, intelligent gaze, I realize who this goddess resembles. Rose, lovely and fearless, leading the way, dismissing qualms, answering questions and showing the path forward. I'm learning from these guides. I've recognized that we need to really pay attention and learn about ourselves from all the various life stages as we experience them. To know ourselves. As the oracle at Delphi advised.

You may be making some progress. Still, you must go further.

Well, I think Leonardo's mirrored labyrinth could surely be a help with that. I see the core of any labyrinth as a kind of Delphic oracle, a way of reflecting upon and ultimately getting to know whowe really are.

There were two other inscriptions on the wall of the temple at Delphi. I don't know why people ignore them. The second piece of advice is 'Nothing in excess.'

I'm reminded that the many-sided view of my aged, over-weight self might well bring this admonition to mind.

The third is the most mysterious. It is simply the letter E, and thereare a great many theories about what this means. I like the one that proposes that Epsilon, the letter E, written as EI, refers to the word "if." If, if, if, if, if...the ever possible.

If is the great enabler. As Touchstone says in *As You Like It*: "*Your If is the only peacemaker; much virtue in If.*"

If is the word that prefaces everything for Rose now. She's still hanging on to life and *if* the swelling in her legs lessens, *if* the antibiotics can control the infection, *if* she can keep food down, *if* they can get a hospital bed and hospice care, *if* all goes well, she can go home.

And, miracle of miracles, the *ifs* do all fall into place. Later on when I phone Rose, I hear real joy in her voice. Her hospital bed has now been set up in her townhouse, facing the doors that lead out to the patio. The night before she came home from the hospital some of her neighbours went out in the moonlight to plant flowers so that she is able to look out on a flourishing courtyard. The light, she says, is astonishing.

I tell her I wish I could be there to help out.

"It was a help simply to have your visit, dear girl. You are a truly wonderful friend. I think I admire you more than anyone I know."

"Really? I don't see why that would be." I've always been the admirer of Rose, not she of me. And what she has reflected back tome, over the years, is my failure to come close to the standard she has set. I have a suspicion that behind admiration there is always a little animosity.

"You don't, do you? Well, one day I'll have to enlighten you."

"Yes. Please. I'd like to understand what you find to admire in me."

"Once you understand," she laughs, "I'll explain."

Another riddle. Rose likes to be mysterious. She reminds me of that great Greek riddler, the Sphinx herself. Another hybrid—a winged creature with the head of a woman and the paws and claws of a lion—the Sphinx lay in wait for travelers at the entrance to thecity of Thebes and posed a riddle to all those who wanted to obtain passage: *Which creature in the morning goes on four feet, at noon on two, and in the evening upon three?* She strangled anyone unable to answer. The word "sphinx," I recall, is related to "sphincter" and means "throttler."

Oedipus escaped by answering correctly as follows: Man, who as a baby crawls on all fours, in maturity walks on two feet, and in old age must lean on a cane. Mortified by defeat, the Sphinx died in the manner of so many of those great Greeks: flinging herself from a cliff. Unlike that demon of destruction, Rose gives and attracts love.

When she first was diagnosed with cancer, she told me that she felt that she was surrounded by a sea of love because her family and friends were all being so supportive. She said this was what has kept her "afloat." But maybe this is a time when, rather than staying afloat, a person needs to let herself go downwards, deeper than she ever has before. Should we who love her help her to do that? Maybe. Maybe not.

Maybe...anything. When I first died, women began to worship me at a sacred place which they called the Grove of Ariadne Aphrodite. They wore wreaths of Artemisia absinthium, a very beautiful plant with silvery green leaves and pale yellow flowers. You call it wormwood. It was the love these women displayed for me that helped me to continue my life as a goddess.

"Are you saying that all you need is love? Like the song says?"

I'm saying that love can see you through a lot of things.

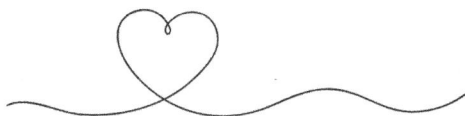

Finding Balance

May is a month of mixtures, but we have no *Maibowle* to celebrate May Day this year. When we first moved to our island home, one of our neighbours introduced us to the German May festivities and the creation of that delicious May libation, the *Maibowle*, which is made by steeping sweet woodruff in a white German wine. Brandy, sparkling wine and strawberries are mixed in to enhance the concoction. This year the month of May is cold, so the sweet woodruff has not yet bloomed. We could make something pretty close to a *Maibowle* without any sweet woodruff, but we have been too busy to celebrate May Day.

I've read that sweet woodruff is slightly poisonous, so it's important not to consume too much of it. The poison in the wine, the mixture of what both sickens and sustains, makes me think about Rose's chemotherapy. I hear from a Toronto acquaintance that it's heartening to see Rose back in her townhouse, surrounded by beautiful flowers. At home, fresh flowers don't present the health hazard they apparently do in hospitals, and certainly they lift Rose'sspirits.

Sometimes it's hard to figure out what's what. Hard to sort out what spirits us from what dispirits. The high spirits from the false spirits. On May Day this year I moderate a panel for an annual mental health forum at which three people speak about their experiences in dealing with psychiatric problems: a father speaks about the perplexing years before and after his son was diagnosed with schizophrenia. A transsexual woman tells us about her history as a man which included marriages she now sees as lesbian relationships. An older man speaks of being in and out of prison until, only a few years ago, he was finally diagnosed and treated for a bipolar disorder.

Each of these people had prevailed along a painful road full of twists and turns and had arrived at a place of hopefulness about what the future holds. Each had come to terms with substance abuse and had renounced alcohol.

"We're drinking far too much these days," I tell Mike. "It's unbecoming in people our age. We must develop moderation."

"I despise moderation. If I can't have excess, I'll choose abstinence," he replies.

But we both know that he will not choose abstinence. Drink is important to him. A few years ago he wrote an essay for *Humanist Perspectives* entitled "On Drink! On Spirit! On Humanity!" In this piece, he claimed that alcohol is the earliest of our sciences and a mark of our civilization. "Alcohol is everything," he wrote, "Drink shapes every activity of humankind."

Now he tells me that alcohol is at the centre of our being, is what gives the oomph to our lives. "As in the Greek word omphalos, which means "the navel," or the "hub." It is what sparks the human spirit." In a private conversation before the May Day conference began, one of the panelists told me that, since he no longer smokes, drinks or uses drugs, his needs are now simple. He requires very little money to survive. When his income assistance was increased a few years ago it occurred to him that he could use the extra money to make a difference for someone else.

"I lost my own family because while I was doing time my wife found someone else and didn't want the children to have anything more to do with me. I thought I'd have to live my life as a childless person, but one day I saw a message about Save the Children, and I realized that was something I could do."

Now he has a little foster daughter in Cambodia, and his face lights up as he speaks of buying colouring books, crayons, and games at the dollar store for her. He sends packages and letters to her and to her parents and is saving a little money every month, trying to accumulate enough for airfare so that in a few years he may be able to meet the child and her family.

"In a few years I'll be getting Old Age Pension cheques," he explains, "so then I'll have plenty of money."

"Wonderful!" Rose says when I call her and recount this story. "A man who has lost and renounced so much, and yet is able to live easily and modestly on the planet in a way that you and I cannot. It makes me think of Gary Snyder's comment that true affluence is not needing anything. Maybe true generosity comes from that sameplace."

On my next labyrinth walk, I ask Ariadne for her thoughts on generosity.

My husband, Dionysus, was generous. I was much happier with him than I could ever have been with Theseus. Theseus was self-absorbed, a very selfish man. Generous men like Dionysus make better partners.

"You were fortunate that he found you."

Yes, my story is actually a very happy one. It was fated to be. In fact, the Fates sang a wedding song foretelling our joyful future, and then Dionysus gave me a magnificent crown, the Corona Borealis, which still lights up your skies at night. I believe it was given to him by Aphrodite.

Ariadne speaks joyfully of her married life, but she downplays the sad parts, such as the death of her winemaker son, Oenopian.

"Did he too commit suicide?"

Some say so. I personally think Perseus killed him.

There are always multiple explanations. I've read one version of her story in which Ariadne died in childbirth and another in which she eventually hanged herself from a tree. Another says she was turned to stone by Perseus. Hard to get these Greek myths straight. Everything Ariadne tells me can be contested in some of the written versions of her story. Whatever the version, there aren't many happy endings.

Just listen to the first aria in Richard Strauss's opera Ariadne auf Naxos *if you want to know how I was feeling when Theseus left me! But then Dionysus appeared and instantly fell in love with me. How could the god of divine intoxication, of wine and revelry fail to lift an unhappy young girl's spirits?*

I take her point. Years ago, I too was young and heartbroken, and then Mike came along and we had such good times together. Bacchanalian times, Dionysian times, with a lot of wine and food and love and laughter.

But surely Bacchanalia is for the young. No matter how much fun we've had, experience teaches us that we must eventually detach ourselves from the things of this world. Pleasures are fleeting and possessions can't satisfy us forever. We have to face losing all the things we have treasured, and in any case our joy in them starts to diminish.

We need to prepare for an end in which youthful diversions are long gone. In the words of Sufi sage Mulla Nasrudin, *One day we will all wear a cloak with no pockets.*

Maybe I should stop worrying about what's yet to come. The women who concocted Bacchic rites to celebrate life and fertility had not much care for the future. I could choose to be like them. It's all about choices, as the addictions people say. And some of the choices are toxic, as we learn to our dismay. "Name your poison," people used to say when they offered you a drink.

Mike says the omphalos can guide us. There's a German band called Ooomph! which has a song about labyrinths: "Left, right, straight ahead, you're in the labyrinth," the song says, "and no-one can tell you who the good and evil are."

The omphalos is one of the sacred objects of the Delphic oracle. Thesecone-shaped stones are worshipped everywhere around the Meditarranean. They represent a channel that allows you to communicate with the gods.

Mike would probably agree that there are connections betweenthe oomph of the wine and the communication with the gods.

The omphalos was named for a stone that existed at the meeting place where Zeus sent two eagles to cross the world. The place where two extremes meet.

So it's a symbol that represents centredness.

It's all a question of balance, my friend.

Because I'm in a research project I have to fill out a questionnaire on my progress each time I go to the cancer clinic for follow-up appointments. I can easily answer the questions about how often my sleep is disturbed (Not Often) and how much support I receive from friends and family (Quite a Bit) but I get stuck on the questions about how hopeful I feel about the future.

"You mean global warming?" I ask. "The food crisis? Overpopulation? Peak oil? Afghanistan?"

"Just focus on your personal health," the young researcher says. "I think that's what they want."

There are some changes in my breast. A little more darkening, more swelling, and a hardening around the area of the scar. I've been wondering about this.

"It's probably scar tissue," my oncologist says. "Or maybe a seroma. I have seen such changes quite a long time after the radiation." She examines my breast closely and says again that it is likely not a problem. "But we'd better do an ultrasound to be sure."

While she's writing the order she looks up at me and says, "It might be best to request that, if they see anything unusual, they do a biopsy right away." I try to interpret from her reactions whether she thinks they will find anything, but her expression is inscrutable.

"It will speed everything up," she says.

"That makes sense," I agree.

I like my oncologist. She's quick and smart. I think she's being honest with me, but I also know that, with cancer, medical people always start by giving you the most hopeful agenda, and then slowly unroll the bad news.

To pass the time while waiting for my ultrasound appointment, I go alone to walk a labyrinth which is very near the hospital. In the parking lot I encounter a long-time colleague from the university. Both retired now, we exchange the usual pleasantries, claiming to be fine until first she acknowledges, "Except, you know, falling apart in all the usual places." We agree that it would be good to get together to "catch up" and know that we probably won't do so.

There are people we like, people we encounter periodically and are always glad to see yet they remain secondary people in our lives. Diana and I would welcome a closer friendship, but events do not bring that about. It is as though we are always just out of reach of each other. But I know we are on the same path and I am glad of her presence.

Making conversation as we step over to the labyrinth, I ask what she knows about the goddess whose name she bears. She tells me that when she was at school, people made fun of her name. Diana being goddess of the hunt, they liked to tell her to go blow her horn. However, whenever she went to Greece, her Greek friends called her Artemis, which she liked much better.

Why, I wonder, do these deities have so many names? It's a question for Ariadne.

34

I know of no goddess named Diana, Ariadne says. *Probably you are referring to Artemis, the protector of wild animals, personification of the moon.*

Diana in Roman times, Artemis in Greek times. Isn't it the same thing? A rose by any other name? Although, as soon as I think this, I realize that no other name would do for Rose.

I'm aware that Ovid and his friends gave Latin names to all our gods and goddesses. They invented stories that simply were not as good as ours. People in your time don't seem to discriminate between the real myths and the Roman versions.

Why does it matter? Ovid, Homer, Virgil, Hesiod. Roman or Greek, they all wrote about Ariadne. The stories are various, and all of them fascinate me.

It's a matter of culture. Our people told stories, sang songs, and the truth was embedded in our voices. Those Roman scribes wanted to write everything down. And they got things wrong.

History does that.

They say it was a time of great change, great turmoil. I suppose it was a bit like your millennium, a time of fear and confusion.

I've been wondering about that. For instance, Ovid's life was between 43 B.C. and 17 A.D. So when he was 40 years old was he was doing the countdown to year zero? 3 years to zero, 2 years to zero, 1 year to zero, and then, ZERO! The point when B.C. changes to A.D.

What was going on in that zero year between B.C. and A.D.?

We never had a word for zero, as a matter of fact. That empty symbol was something that came much later. We concerned ourselves with presence, not absence.

Diana and I meet again at the door of the hospital and walk to the waiting room together but, once there, we take seats on opposite sides of the room, turn to our books, and wait for our numbers to be called. Each of us has worked in hospitals in the past, she as a nurse and I as a social worker, so we're familiar with the routine here. We understand the necessary barriers that exist between the well and the ill, the professionals and the lay people, and we settle into our current roles as patients.

Years ago, when I first worked in hospitals everyone wore white lab coats, even the office staff, which highlighted our status as officially healthy people. Nowadays the staff have large, plasticized photo I.D. hanging from their necks or swinging from their belts alongside their keys, suggesting not just caretakers but jailers. There's a fair amount of time involved in taking a number, registering at the desk, moving to a secondary waiting room, sitting around while X-rays are located and examined and so, not surprisingly, patients will go off to get coffee, to go to the washroom, or just to stretch their legs. Now the staff call out again and again, for patients who have wandered off during one of the stages of awaiting medical treatment.

"He's over there...you just missed him...you'll catch him com- ing around the corner...maybe he went that way," the other patients explain. It's a bit of a labyrinth here too, I think, and just at that moment the large, cheerful, Native man across from me smiles and says the only word I've heard him say: carousel. It's just the right image for the way I'm feeling. Not really a labyrinth, nor a maze, nor a roller coaster, but a carousel with its predictable ups and downs and endless circling. Endless until one day, at last, it will stop. That's the name of the game.

There are always moments when time seems to stop. What you might call the zero points. But then, after awhile, it all moves forward again.

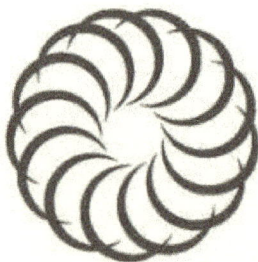

Transformations

The day after the ultrasound appointment, Mike and I take off to spend a few days visiting family and staying a few nights at a meditative retreat which features a stone and turf labyrinth on a hillside overlooking a lake. On the way we stop at the studio of our friend Al McWilliams and our attention is caught by some unusual images: huge photographs of worms, images that Mike says he finds exciting.

I find them disturbing but also affecting. "Black gold," Al laughs. "These ones are photographs of my compost."

The images have now been turned into several signs, as part of a larger public art exhibition, with the text "Development Permit Application."

"Many people seem to be discomfited by the worms," Al says. "Maybe it reminds them of internal organs or their own mortality—the fact that they will one day end up becoming worm food." It's true that a lot of development takes place underground, and maybe we should pay more attention to that.

"I guess your images could also be seen as celebrating transformation," I say. "The garden offers an inspiring metaphor for our lives. Birth and rebirth and so on. Continuity."

"I do think of them as transformers," Al says, "and not just because of their valuable work in the compost. They themselves are always changing. At times they look spare and calligraphic, and at other times they are densely intertwined and teeming with activity." "I find the worms cheerful," Mike says, "and it's satisfying to think that in the end we all turn into compost. You could view the developmental stages of human aging as parallel to the experience of planting, fertilizing, and maturing in the way that plants develop as they grow, change and ripen and decompose."

We drive through low rolling hills that are now covered with wildflowers. The landscape is open, expansive, sunny and hot, and in parts almost desert-like. Throughout the drive we see signs of the pine beetle epidemic we've read about: discoloured, dead or dying trees, and government signs about the programs to prevent further destruction. I've read that carbon dioxide emissions created the warmer environment that supports the increase of pine beetles and also that the death of the trees from the infestations will dramatically increase carbon dioxide emissions in these forests. The red-tinged trees are beautiful despite their disease, but it's depressing to consider the future of the forests.

As the rising road becomes hard-packed dirt, we see a sign that marks the driveway to the retreat centre which is home to an eleven-circuit outdoor rock labyrinth. The centre's founder had constructed the labyrinth in the midst of a field of Ponderosa pines. We'd been advised that the labyrinth was greatly transformed when the trees that were an integral part of the original pathway were destroyed by the pine beetle infestation and chopped down, but I was not prepared for the extent of the damage I see when we begin to walk the labyrinth.

At first I'm shocked by the stumps inside the stone circle and the heaps of ashes from the branches that had been burned, yet at the same time I appreciate the wonderful spaciousness and the uninterrupted view of the lake. Even now, among the stumps that remain, I'm aware of the presences that no longer occupy the space. I can see that the trees would have provided shade and shadow, obstacles, challenges and support.

The centre's leader tells us that when she first came to this hillside property, it had become, as vacant rural properties often do, a resting place for automobile corpses.

"When we were building the labyrinth we had to remove a number of old cars that had been left to rust," she explains, "and people used to say that they felt a sense of gratitude from the trees as they walked among them."

She says she grieved for the lost trees and for a time, when they were first gone, she was unable to walk the labyrinth. At first she thought it was dead but then began to see it as resurrected, with a new shape and a new presence.

Inspired by a labyrinth in a labyrinth which she thought of as the circle of birth and death, she created a similar cycle in her labyrinth by placing black and white stones at the centre. Life and death intermingled were part of the original design and the juxtaposition is now intensified through the presence of the stumps and ashes mixed with the new growth of shrubs and flowers. The pine beetles lived on the living tree and then the trees died. The beetles were destroyed and the infested branches were burnt to ashes. From the ashes came fresh ground for new growth.

Also in the centre chamber, surprisingly, are dozens of tiny cherry pits from the nearby orchard, along with the white and black stones that Flo has set there. Those cherry pits invite thoughts of origins, beginnings, tiny things that may be the germ of great creations. Hints or reminders of the many projects, large and small, that we've neglected or not yet started. And also of what has been consumed.

One of the unique aspects of this setting is the sense of apprehension we experience in the labyrinth. This hillside setting requires the walker to pay more attention than in one laid out on a church hall or gymnasium floor or in a city garden. The ground is uneven, irregular stones defining the path, and the stumps remaining from the pines to be stepped over or stepped around. The most striking obstacle to being transported from the here and now to a faraway realm of pure thought is the slope of the ground. Moving uphill in the direction of the entrance, we are bent forward, pushing a bit, labouring a little. As we circle and move downhill, we lean back, bracing ourselves.

The surroundings are splendid, but the landscape is dry, dry, dry. I find myself thinking of the arid background described in Sheila Watson's novel *The Double Hook*, a parched landscape in which the grasses and creeks have dried up, and dust and death are everywhere. Here too, the light and the dark are juxtaposed.

"When you fish for glory, you catch the darkness too," Watson writes. Maybe the reverse is also true. The wildflowers that have sprung up within the dark ashes of Flo's labyrinth are surprising and glorious. I find myself thinking about the story of Persephone. When she was abducted, her mother, Demeter, caused the springs to run dry, the vegetation to languish, and the land to be made barren and infertile. Once her daughter was returned to her, the land came back to life and was again fertile and fruitful. Death, rebirth, and transformation were everywhere there, as they are here.

"I've come up with some new words to describe the writing of the landscape: 'toporeography' and 'toporeopathy,' to describe the writing about a place, and the relations of illness to a place," Mike announces, as we pack our bags.

"And I have a better one," I tell him. "Mine is 'toporeification,' making the land sacred by building a labyrinth. Or maybe that should be 'topodeification.'"

After making visits to our family, we begin the drive home, stopping at a labyrinth painted on the pavement space that lies between two churches. Because today is a statutory holiday, the heavy gate in the chain link fence is bolted shut, so we are unable to enter. The setting for this labyrinth is not as beautiful as some, yet it is another labyrinth in the world, and I'm glad to see that there is such a proliferation of these patterned spaces. I think how the leader of the labyrinth we'd just left had stood at her doorway, pointing to a mass of grey-headed weeds, and exclaiming, "Look at that lovely bunch of dandelions," she said. "They're just waiting for the wind to lift them!" Labyrinths are spreading in much the same way. It's an inspiring phenomenon.

The brief holiday has been restful and I'm grateful for the tranquil peace and beauty of countryside, but as we near home my thoughts darken. I think of the dandelions, the pine beetles, we humans, all of us swarming, spreading, multiplying. Destroying, devastating. The world appears to be a spiritual wasteland, with humans the greatest plague, the worst infestation.

Decades ago, Jonas Salk, the man who developed the polio vaccine, pointed out that life on earth would soon disappear if all the insects disappeared, whereas if all the humans disappeared other species would flourish as never before.

My little granddaughter was right when, at the age of three, she announced to a large group, "There are too many humans here. Would the humans please leave now?" She has always thought that animals were a better bet.

The future of our planet looks bleak, but when we return home, my doctor phones with good news. The ultrasound came back clear. I am spared. For the moment.

Things change. At the darkest moment, the light can still return. Transformation is always possible. We have the seasons as a reminder of that.

Successful Aging

To celebrate my renewed lease on life, I take Mike to see a lovely labyrinth on a nearby island. A tile path lined with upended stones leads the way to this classical, seven-circuit left-handed Cretan gravel labyrinth which offers a view of the ocean through the surrounding tall trees, ferns and rhododendrons. It's a brilliantly sunny day with a slight breeze that sets wind chimes tinkling in the tall trees.

The creator of this island built it for his wife in memory of her sister who had died of cancer a few years earlier. At the entrance to the labyrinth is his interpretation of the meaning of the labyrinth: "Life is a labyrinth—a long, winding pathway full of experiences and challenges that eventually doubles back on itself to end at the place where it first began."

That feels true. We seem to go forward and then events that weencounter take us back to earlier times. As T.S. Eliot wrote:

> We shall not cease from exploration
> And the end of all our exploring
> Will be to arrive where we started
> And know the place for the first time.

At the centre of this labyrinth is a tile representation of the yin yang symbol and a memorial inscription. I am moved both by the experience of walking this pleasant path and by the inscription on the tile: *in loving memory*. It could refer to loving the memory of a person or to being in the state of loving memory. It might refer to the love of memory itself. Whatever the case, this tribute gives the labyrinth a beautiful heart.

Memory can be a kind of monster that we confront as we age, one that yields recollections that haunt us, shadows that must be explored at the depths of one's being. When I was at the previous retreat centre, I was given a prayer adapted by Jim Cotter which asks for "a candle of the spirit" to lead down to "the deeps" of being:

Show me the hidden things, the creatures of my dreams,
the storehouse of forgotten memories and hurts.
Take me down to the spring
of my life and tell me
my nature and my name.

I know that I must confront my own shadows as part of learning to accept change, decay and death, but it's hard to face some memories, especially those which make me feel guilt and shame at my own behaviour. "Who knows what evil lurks in the hearts of men?" an old radio program from my youth routinely asked. "The Shadow knows," was the answer.

Today my question for Ariadne is, "What can I do to prepare for the end of times?" I'm reading Jung's *Memoirs, Dreams, Reflections*, published shortly before his death. He wrote "I try to see the line which leads through my life into the world, and out of the world again." That's the labyrinth, and I think the hardest part is seeing the way out. That's why I'm sometimes afraid to go into that inner territory. Afraid that I'll never get out.

What does the labyrinth teach you about that, my friend?

"The path that leads you in is the path that leads you out. I know that. It doesn't stop the fear."

Remember what that Roman fellow said: Solvitur ambulando.

"St. Augustine. It is solved by walking."

Yes. Keep on walking, my friend.

It would be heartening to imagine that the weakness of age will strengthen us and make us wise. That's what Cicero proposes in his *DeSenectute*, arguing that old age is in many ways superior to youth. For example, he says, the steersman of a boat who sits quietly while young men hurry up and down gangways performs the more valuable task.

But I'm not sure that the pleasures of the mind compensate for the debilitation of the body. "Healthy mind, healthy body— take your pick!" was a slogan I heard as a young person and, although I didn't take good care of my physical health, there is no doubt in my mind what my choice would be now. The best I can do is follow Ariadne's advice and keep on walking.

"Walking the labyrinth is helping me to face the reality of aging and death," I tell Mike. "The labyrinth is leading me to some different things. Who knows what I might take up next? Many creative people do some of their most interesting work late in life. Bach, Yeats, Coleridge, Stravinsky, Picasso. Just a few examples."

Erik Erikson says the seventh stage of psychological development is the achievement of generativity versus stagnation. The eighth and final stage is integrity versus despair. An experience of integrity occurswhen a person reviews her life and feels positive about how it has all gone. Otherwise, she feels despair. But it seems to me that the final sense of integrity is also still connected with generativity. It has to do with participating in the world, caring for the next generation and "passing on" whatever one has to contribute. Continuing to believe that there is a future, even when we know the damage that is being done by human behaviour, continuing pollution and climate change.

Everywhere I turn I see fear of aging. For my birthday recently, Mike gave me a perfume called *Ageless*, described in English as "anti-age perfume," in French as *eau jeunesse*. I'd told him I wanted a perfume with a grapefruit scent, and *Ageless* combines the essence of pink grapefruit, mango, pomegranate, jasmine and musk. It's lovely.

The box in which the perfume is packaged says the scent is designed to make you smell younger and claims that "Research has proven that men around women who use *Ageless* anti-age perfume believe them to be at least eight years younger!" I wonder how this research was conducted. Did they line up a lot of incredibly old women, women older than one could possibly imagine, and spray them all over with "Ageless," then ask the men to guess their age?

"Ninety-four," they might say. "Ninety-six," perhaps. But who could have guessed that the women were actually a hundred and two, a hundred and four?

Going out to a dinner party on the night of my birthday, I wore the perfume. Everyone liked it, men and women. When I explained its purpose, they agreed that it had a nice, light, youthful scent, but I doubt they were confused about my actual age. The next morning,while I was visiting a neighbour, Mike dropped the perfume, which I'd foolishly left on a kitchen counter, and cracked the bottle on our tile floor. When I returned home he apologized briefly but was very proud of how he responded to this event, by pouring the remaining perfume into a cocktail shaker.

"When you pour perfume out of a cocktail shaker, you need to pour it into something like a martini glass," I point out. "The mouth is too wide to use it as a perfume bottle. It won't work." I demonstrate by pouring some onto my wrists and thus splashing a good deal onto the floor, which instantly made our whole house smell younger!

Such events will happen more and more frequently. My absent-mindedness in leaving the perfume on the kitchen counter. His, in finding such an inappropriate solution. But we carry on.

"I need fresh adventures and meaningful purpose in my life. I want to live, live, live until I die," I tell Mike. "Lots of old people are learning new things. Look at Grandma Moses. She was almost eighty when she took up painting and she continued to paint until she was a hundred." I carry on with my arguments about the importance of making a contribution, doing work that leaves behind a legacy of some sort.

Once again, Mike has the last word, and once again it's Woody Allen. "I don't want to achieve immortality through my work," he says, "I want to achieve it through not dying."

Mortals die. That's the way it's always been.

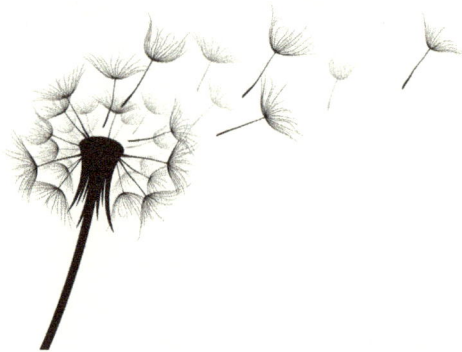

Daedalus Revisited

One of the most interesting modern labyrinths we discovered at a retreat centre not far from where we live is a Chalice labyrinth. Designed by Robert Peach, it is in the classical tradition but has the addition of the Chartres-style "labyrs," the double-ax shapes, at the turning points.

For Minoans, the double-ax was a symbol of the Goddess, and it continues today to serve as an important feminist symbol. Sometimes the double-ax is seen as a wand, topped with a butterfly, a happy image. In addition to housing the Minotaur, the labyrinth served as a dancing floor for the Goddess. In the *Iliad*, Homer describes the labyrinth as being home to tumbling and singing and "merry and tinkling feet." I somehow doubt that the seven youths and seven maidens who were sent to Knossos on those nonennial pilgrimages were dancing as they made their way towards death.

The shape of the chalice design gives a strong central focus, and the large centre offers a greater meditative space than many other labyrinth structures. Describing the sacred geography of the design, Peach refers to the three left circuits representing heaven meeting the four right circuits which represent earth, at the entrance of the chalice, which represents the "Christ Consciousness." Peach has shared his design freely, providing directions for labyrinth builders, and the original design has now attracted many variations, of which this labyrinth is one.

Constructed with dwarf English boxwood and rock, it has a refreshing feeling of newness and originality. The shrubs are small, which gives a sense that the labyrinth is both settling in and growing around us.

Inside the retreat centre we are shown a number of finger labyrinths that have been made by Bill Godden for use at pilgrimages and workshops.

"Could I purchase one of these?" I ask.

"Bill won't sell his labyrinths," I'm told. "He'll only give them away. And he'd want you to have one, so take your pick."

This spirit of generosity is something I find remarkable in labyrinth people. There seems to be an open heartedness connected with the love of labyrinths.

I've heard that even when people intend to build a labyrinth on their own property for their private use, things often change for them in the process of building it. Often when the labyrinth evolves, the builder stops suddenly and says, "People are going to want to walk this labyrinth. I'll have to open it up."

Bill Godden is a good example of this generosity. He describes himself as a "labyrinth hobbyist," who makes his labyrinths out of recycled wood and then gives them away to friends who are labyrinth facilitators. But he won't consider selling them. He's been fascinated by the patterns of the labyrinth ever since the day on which he first saw the labyrinth located outside the Vancouver School of Theology at the University of British Columbia. Working with ordinary hand and machine tools, Bill has created hundreds of finger labyrinths with more than twenty different designs. His creativity makes me think of him as a modern-day Daedalus.

The labyrinths are various and all so beautiful that I find it difficult to make a decision, but finally I choose a Santa Rosa Labyrinth©, which says #616 on the back. Bill has said that he intends to create a thousand finger labyrinths and so he numbers each of them.

This Santa Rosa Labyrinth is a seven-circuit, neo-medieval design created by Dr. Lea Goode-Harris in 1997. What interests me most about this pattern is the small open space in the fourth path. Dr. Goode-Harris says this emerged when she lined up the entrance with the path into the center. As a separate sacred space which is never entered, it can hold one's symbols or hopes. It can be viewed from all four directions and is described by Goode-Harris as the "heart space."

Lea Goode-Harris describes her life work as bringing "an inquisitive heart to educating, designing, making, and researching labyrinths."

As a poet, writer and mixed media artist, she has worked with others to create a number of traditional and contemporary labyrinths in various settings, including the construction of a 22-foot

Santa Rosa Labyrinth at her own home. Lea offers talks and workshops at conferences and educational institutions, and she has created a charming little portable finger labyrinth for children which features a ladybug finding her way home.

Tracing a finger labyrinth can be a pleasant and accessible form of meditation. Finger labyrinths are portable and easy to use at all times, and it's possible to pace your walk at different speeds, accordingto your mood. There's a reassuring feel to the smooth wooden edges of Bill Godden's finger labyrinth. I've been told that walking a finger labyrinth seven times before going to bed can help you to get a good sleep. It's worth a try. Lea Goode-Harris tells me that when she awakens in the middle of the night and cannot sleep she walks one of two labyrinths (the Santa Rosa Labyrinth or Hopi design) in her mind and is usually back asleep before reaching the center.

There are many virtual finger labyrinths available on the internetthese days. Grace Cathedral in San Francisco offers online labyrinth walks, and there's also a lovely little online walk you can take by using your mouse to lead a small white dove in and out of a Chartres- style labyrinth. These online labyrinths provide a useful resource for many people, but if I am not going to walk the path with my feet, I prefer to feel that at least my fingers are touching an actual path.

The empty space in the Santa Rosa Labyrinth reminds me of something that I puzzle over until suddenly I remember the "slip room" a friend described encountering when she stayed in an old home in St. John's, Newfoundland. The tiny room, she said, was used only when people were being born or dying. Entering life or leaving it. The enclosed space on the Santa Rosa Labyrinth is also its own realm. A separate place, a place of the heart, a slip room. As my fingers walk Bill's labyrinth, I pause to reflect on that empty space. The hidden room. A place of mystery.

Irish writer and social philosopher Charles Handy says that one is meant in life to discover a hidden part of oneself in order to learn who we can be and what we can ultimately become. He keeps a small white stone on his desk to remind him of this purpose, and he refers to the mysterious verse in the Book of Revelations in the Bible, a verse which says: "To the one who prevails," the Spirit says, "I will give a white stone…on which is written a name, which shall be known only to the one who receives it."

Jim Cotter's poem about discovering "my nature and my name" echoes the same point. The search, then, is to discover who one really is at the deepest level—the self one doesn't yet know. The emerging self. And surely acknowledging the better self that one could become, with effort, goes side by side with recognizing the worst in oneself, the monster within. The Minotaur at the centre.

Gernot Candolini writes about a Mirror Maze in the English town of Wookey Hole. Above one of the mirrors in the maze is an engraving that says, "This is the Minotaur." The ultimate confrontation with the monster lies simply in seeing oneself. But it would be even more shocking to face oneself in the labyrinth that Leonardo da Vinci designed, one in which you would see your reflection from all angles. To face all the dark sides of oneself at once! As in the story about Perseus making the Gorgons look at their own reflections in his shield, which promptly turned them into stone. One's own reflection can be dangerous.

Everything is dangerous. When you accept that, the dark places lose their terror. Consider Daedalus, locked up in the labyrinth that he himself had constructed. He saw the sky, and so he set out to create a set of wings.

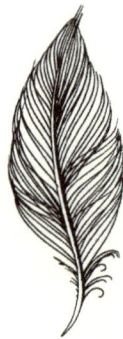

Defining Life Realistically

Defining life realistically is another of Jung's tasks for successful aging, but it's hard to do this. Just when you think you have a handle on things, everything changes. Your life happens slowly—and then all of a sudden everything is quick. You turn your head, turn a page on the calendar, and in just an instant you are facing a new scenario.

Rose is now in a hospice facility, which is a good thing because even with the help of caregivers she could no longer live alone. I go to Toronto again to see how she is faring and, when I arrive, I find her sleeping soundly. I'm surprised by how old she has become. Of course, her vigor could not have been expected to last forever, yet it's a shock to see her now, so emaciated and bent over. Her face, still handsome, lacks the vitality which once distinguished her. The cancer is now almost everywhere and her pain is acute. She's stopped colouring her hair and wears no make-up.

I leave her asleep and walk down to the labyrinth at the church of the Holy Trinity. It's a cool afternoon, so I walk briskly around the stone curves of the path. Today, as usual, I ask the ultimate questions of Ariadne. *What is the way out? Where does it lead?*

More specifically, what can I say to Rose, who sees no curve in her path? What she sees is a straight line from birth to death, nothing beyond. Not for her Blake's "New Jerusalem."

> I give you the end of a golden string;
>> Only wind it into a ball,
> It will lead you in at Heaven's gate,
>> Built in Jerusalem's wall.

Just keep walking, my friend. Trust the path you have chosen. Your friend will follow her own course.

When I return to the care facility, I find Rose awake and in a cheerful mood, wanting to hear about everything I've been doing.

"I've come from the labyrinth," I tell her, "where I did a crane dance in your honour."

"Show me."

I bend over, one arm forward and one back, and try to hop in a circle around her bed.

"I need more room," I tell her. "I'll show you out in the hall later. It's a good space for the crane dance. The dance is the *geranos*, the Greek word for 'crane,' and it's used in courtship as well as in war. The Spartans liked dancing almost as much as they did combat."

"Love and war. They wanted to make love *and* war," Rose mutters, thinking of the slogans from earlier times when we attended peace marches together. Rose has championed social and political causes since her adolescence and even now, confined to a care facility, her interest in these outside activities has not waned.

I think of Simone de Beauvoir's argument in *The Coming of Age*, that old age must be a time of creative and meaningful projects and relationships with others. Above all else, she proposed, old age must be not a time of boredom but a time of continuous political and social action. It's no longer possible for Rose to engage in social action but she does keep up with current events and the activities of her friends, and she inquires with real interest about a labyrinth workshop I recently led.

"Fascinating," Rose says, "tell me all about it."

"What people liked best were the finger labyrinths I gave them." I tell her about Bill Godden's labyrinths and about his insistence on giving them away rather than selling them. She's delighted by such generosity, as I knew she would be.

"How do they work, these finger labyrinths? Do you believe they have an actual purpose?"

"Some people say that tracing the pattern into the centre and out again can help you sleep."

"It would be better than these," she gestures towards the array of medication on her night table, "if it really worked."

"I'll send you one," I promise. How could I not have thought to bring one with me? I'm conscious that there's not a lot of time, and my thoughtlessness pains me. I remember, and foresee, an accumulation of careless behaviour and lost opportunities.

"What else did you do in your workshop?"

"Mike came for part of the session and talked about what he called the three great inventions of Daedalus. I only wanted him to tell the labyrinth story, actually. I'd just brought him in for a change of voice, a bit of variety, but I should have known he'd go off on a tangent of his own. He started by drawing three symbols on the white-board: a pair of trousers, a double-headed axe, and a set of wings."

Rose gestures for me to help her to sit up and asks for details. I tell her about Mike's notion that Daedalus had these three significant achievements: facilitating trans-species sexuality, transcending the rules of physics, and challenging the laws of gravity.

"The trousers represent the wooden cow that Daedalus built for Passiphae so that she could attract the passions of the white bull for which she lusted. It was kind of a cow-suit, he said, covered with a pelt. Mike says it was like a pair of wooden trousers with a flap, a trapdoor that permitted entry from the bull's member. This first feat was significant because it resulted in trans-species copulation."

"Cowsuit," Rose says. "I'll remember that."

I continue with Daedalus's second feat which Mike symbolized as the double axe, the labrys pattern which indicates the turns on the path of the Chartres labyrinth.

"The labrys is also a symbol of feminist power," Rose reminds me, "and of lesbianism. And the butterfly design is also about transformation."

"Mike meant it to symbolize the labyrinth and he says this second feat of Daedalus, commanded by King Minos, defied the laws of physics in that the labyrinth permitted entry and exit for the people who fed or cared for the Minotaur, but did not allow the Minotaur or his victims to escape."

"One of those puzzling paradoxes," Rose concedes.

"The third great achievement, symbolized by the wings, was defying the law of gravity. That was when Daedalus collected feathers and fashioned wings for himself and his son, Icarus, to escape the labyrinth in which Minos had imprisoned them."

"I thought it was a tower."

"Sometimes a tower, sometimes a labyrinth," I say. "There's always another version of the story. And there's always mystery. They're often contradictory. Inexplicable."

"But the wings worked. As long as you didn't get too close to the sun."

"Yes," I say, remembering how I once thought of Rose herself as the sun, and noting that she seems less dangerous now than in the past. "They both flew out, but Icarus forgot Daedalus's warning and flew so close to the sun that his wings melted and he plummeted into the ocean."

I'm glad I made the decision to spend this week with Rose. For the few days we have together we talk intensely about everything important in our lives—husbands, children, books, food. About who and what we love.

"I know a lot about love," Rose claims. She has a dreamy expression, a wistful smile.

"You should write a book about it," I tell her. "You could call it "What I Know About Love: A Great Deal.""

"I've thought of it," she says, "but there isn't time. Did I ever tell you my theory of love?"

"I didn't know you had a theory. But I knew you had a lot of experience."

"My theory is based on experience. I'll explain it to you. There are three levels of love. The first is when you take intense delight in the very existence of that person, in simply knowing that he is alive in the world, being just as he is." She pauses, smiling at the thought of this love.

"The second is when that person makes you happy. When he satisfies all your needs. When the two of you are entirely in harmony with each other." We exchange knowing glances, having had many conversations about such an idyllic state and having each experienced the disappointment of seeking deep intimacy from men who need to guard their emotions. I'm now happily resigned to the impossibility of getting apples from a man who has only oranges to offer, but I don't know that Rose ever accepted Pierre's limitations. Even after his death, she railed about the fact that he withheld his deepest feelings from her.

"The third type of love is what most people have after a long marriage, and it's simply a residue of what was once there. Merely memories. Shared experiences. That is not enough."

She catches her breath and coughs for several moments, then reaches for her painkillers. I refill her glass of ginger ale.

"The one that's really important," she says at last, "is the first type. It's great if you have all three, but it's the first that matters. You've got to have that pleasure in the other's existence. It's essential. I had that with Pierre."

When she drifts off into sleep again, I sit for a few moments by the window and look out on the leafy garden. Rose's world has grown small. This room, pleasant enough for a facility of this sort, is very different from the spacious homes in which I have visited her, though some of the familiar essentials are here. She's brought with her a small oil painting of the Bridge of Sighs. On the side table is an array of little carvings, ivory jungle elephants and tiny china creatures. The windowsill is home to a pretty silver bird next to three large wooden angels. I wonder if these objects will lose their charm when Rose is dead. What seem like treasures during one's lifetime can appear to be rubbish once their owner has left.

There's a small CD player in her room and I've brought some music for Rose to listen to: Rostropovich playing the Bach Cello Suites, the Faure Requiem with John Rutter and the Cambridge Singers. The two pieces of music I would like to hear when I am dying. I settle in to listen to the Bach, concentrating on the winding phrases and systematic patterns—not unlike the labyrinth—and the peculiar structure of the suites. There are the five constant movements—Prelude, Allemande, Courante, Sarabande and Gigue—but the penultimate movement changes. Sometimes a Minuet, a Bourrée, or a Gavotte. I'm thinking about the penultimate as always being a turning point, when suddenly I hear Rose calling out to me.

"What a terrible dream! I was in a cowsuit, it was Mike's story about Daedalus. It was terrifyingly awful…a long, oblong wooden box, and I couldn't get out."

I expect in our minds we're both seeing the image of a coffin, but neither of us speaks of that interpretation.

"I knew it was a cowsuit," Rose said, "because of the little flap. I guess I was dreaming of that little flap because I needed to urinate. And," she turns to me and smiles, "I really do, so could you please help me to get up?"

After she is settled back in her bed again, Rose tells me she wants to sleep, but asks me to leave something for her to drink. I pour apple juice into a delicate, miniature brandy glass with a slender stem that she has brought from home because it's an easier size for her to lift now that she's so weak.

"Poor Daedalus," she says. "He loved his son and grieved for him. He named the island of Icaria after him."

"Love isn't always easy. Nor is flying." I know there is more I should say, but what? Rose, as always, is directing the conversation. "Do you know," she muses, "I once saw a sign for a travel agency called Icarus Tours?"

"How frightening! Who would travel with such a crew?"

That's the kind of trip I'm about to take." She smiles to make sure it is a joke. "You go back and walk your labyrinth now. I'm going to sleep."

"It breaks my heart to leave you," I say, and we hold each other for several minutes, not wanting to say goodbye. We both know that this may be our last visit. The end is near.

"That's OK," Rose grins through her tears. "If your heart isn't broken, you don't know anything about love. Don't even know you have a heart."

On the way out of the lodge I encounter a tiny gnome of an old woman who is hobbling through the corridors with the aid of a walker. Gesturing for me to come closer she says, "These corridors are amazing. It's like an endless path, isn't it? You can go round and round and come back to the same place."

It's a quiet time now, the late afternoon hiatus between teatime and dinner, and the facility is silent but for the two of us.

"Look at those closed doors," the old woman says, "You know, behind every one of those doors, there's a story. Some days I just stop and try to listen to the stories. I say to myself, 'I wonder what the story is behind that door.' You understand what I'm saying?"

She gives me a quizzical look, as though asking for approval. "Yes, I'm sure you are right," I respond, "and that's a good way of looking at things."

"Yes," she agrees, nodding her head, "and then other days I ask myself why I don't just go and slit my fucking wrists…"

I'm taken aback by her vehemence, but she looks up at me with a crafty smile, stops walking for a moment, pats my hand, and continues to speak.

"And then I say to myself, 'Oh, just shut up, you silly old bitch and be grateful for what you've got.'"

I laugh along with her, but her words echo in my mind as I begin my last walk at the Holy Trinity labyrinth. The sky is darkening and I'm alone here, except for a few shadowy figures skirting across the courtyard. I've come here for a sense of closure yet am coming away with the mutterings of an old madwoman.

Pay attention to what you hear. The spoken stories are always the truest.

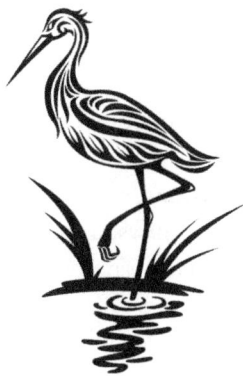

Conducting a Life Review

Surely it is synchronicity when, just as I'm considering another of Jung's tasks for successful aging, that of "conducting a life review," I receive the gift of a book called *Time Traveler* by physicist Dr. Ronald L. Mallett. On the flyleaf my friend has written, simply, "I read this and thought of you."

Why would this book have made him think of me? Certainly, an autobiographical account of a scientist's lifelong research into time travel is not one that would usually appeal to me, yet it is timely. And fascinating. Mallett tells an affecting story of his childhood dream of building a time machine. He wanted to travel back in time to see his dead father and perhaps save him from his premature death. In telling the story, beginning with his discovery of the Classics comic book version of H.G.Wells' *The Time Machine*, Mallet traces and explains the theories that helped him to develop his own theory of time travel.

I have vivid memories of that Classic comic from my own childhood and, although I can't follow all the theoretical material, I love the elegance of the equations Mallet cites and the potential of concepts such as "closed loops of time" and "parallel universes." One of the ideas that most interests me is the parallel-worlds theory developed by Oxford physicist David Deutsch which states that "at every possible decision point, the universe splits into different parallel branches."

It reminds me of T.S. Eliot's poem "Little Gidding" in which he says that what might have been remains "a perpetual possibility" in the world of speculation. The might-have-been, all the might-have-beens, do not disappear but travel along with us. All those split-off branches are part of us. To conduct a life review, then, it makes sense to think about and come to terms with the "might-have-beens" in one's life. I idly trace the winding path of Bill Godden's finger labyrinth, skirting around the empty space. Suddenly I remember a piece of sculpture I'd seen at a gallery when I first went to Montreal, over 40 years ago. It was a glass box with a head on top and wings on each side, but the box itself was empty. Like the circle that creates a zero. The image has stayed with me, that head and those wings, fastened to a vacant space.

My life often felt like that in my younger days, even though so many paths were open to me. So many possibilities. "Where might I otherwise have been led?" This is the question I keep in my mind as I walk the labyrinth. What if I hadn't quit school when I was seventeen, and had gone straight on to university instead? Or, what if, having quit school, I'd gone directly to Paris as I'd originally planned? What if the man I first loved had not taken his own life? What life might we have had together? What if I hadn't married Mike? Hadn't quit all those jobs? The alternate worlds fan out before me. What if I'd been successful in my one abortive suicide attempt? That one, at least, is easily answered.

Diana is at the labyrinth again. I didn't intend to meet her here but, as always, when I find myself walking alongside her in a parallel circuit I'm happy to be in her company. There are many similarities in the twists our separate lives have taken. We've grown up at the same time, had the same kind of work, faced the same illness. Diana has a tranquility that I admire. She is calm, grounded and optimistic. Like Rose, she shows me a possible path through the days ahead, serving as a kind of double for me, a parallel life.

There are always doublings in the labyrinth. The way in and the way out. The double-sided axe. The wings. The mirroring of oneself in so many surprising ways. The light and the dark. Jung and his shadow. The *doppelganger*. At the labyrinth's centre it comes to me that, despite all the twists and turns, my life could not have been different than it has been.

Joseph Campbell, the great mythologist, said, "We must be willing to get rid of the life we planned, so as to have the life that is waiting for us." But I feel that I didn't plan anything, nor did I cast off any plan. However, whatever might have been, this is the world I chose myself, decision after decision. Or non-decision. I need to acknowledge this reality, no matter how much I might yearn for those alternative lives.

I see you have your friend Artemis with you again.

"Diana. Her name is Diana."

Another version of the same story. Aren't you learning anything from your labyrinthine studies?

Ariadne finds me a slow student. I find her a quixotic teacher. "I thought I was making progress."

It's one thing to take responsibility for your choices. But you must also learn to accept that, whatever you chose, those other worlds, those paths you didn't take, have their own reality. Do not wonder what if...accept that they have their place. Look at all the different stories there are about my life and choices.

I have looked at a number of those stories. Plutarch, Hesiod, Ovid and later historians all tell her tale differently. Pregnant by Theseus, dying in childbirth, hanging herself, killed by Artemis. Or happily married to Dionysus, having many children by him, and dying much later in life. In most versions of her life, she is portrayed as a tragic heroine, a victim who came to a sad ending.

The stories are contradictory, so much so that some writers propose that there were at least two Theseuses and two Ariadnes living out our different lives. Look at all the names people have given me: Ariadne, Arianhod, Aryana. All living alternate lives on different continents at different times. It's perfectly possible that we have multiple lives, my friend. But my own version is that Dionysus and I married and lived happily ever after.

"Parallel universes."

There are many mysteries in our world, and in yours.

I remain for a time at the place of mystery, the last petal of the labyrinth, contemplating parallel universes, the curving path and the comfort it gives me. It pleases me that the design is ancient, and I can persuade myself that I'm connecting with a parallel universe from several centuries ago, a time when people walked the Chartres labyrinth. Perhaps they too were deliberating on the meaning of their lives, on questions that are very old and remain unanswered.

Dr. Lauren Artress points out that, while there may not be a direct connection between the labyrinth and the cathedral school which was at the Chartres Cathedral from the sixth to the twelfth centuries, the labyrinth is based on the knowledge of the scholars of the School of Chartres. The central questions asked by these scholars, she says, had to do with healing the soul, healing the planet, healing the body social, questions which still challenge us today.

How is it that more than eight centuries later, we're no closer to answering these questions? Despite our vast numbers, human-kind grows no wiser.

The last time I took Charlotte to a labyrinth, she asked me why sometimes there is a flower at the centre and sometimes just a circle. I told her that I thought the rose was always present within the circle, even if it was invisible, and that I liked to think of what the six petals represent when I am in the centre. Going clockwise around the labyrinth, the petals symbolize mineral, vegetable, ani-mal, human, angel or mystery. I explained that I liked to stand in the place of mystery where I could ask questions about all the things I don't understand. Charlotte decided she would divide her time between the animal petal and the angel petal.

"Animals and angels, those are the ones I like," she announces, running back and forth between the two and skirting around the human realm.

That gets me thinking about hybrids again, and the connections between the six petals. I like the idea of hybrid art forms that mix media, or cross genres, or bridge different cultures, sometimes creat-inga new form that benefits from both gaining and losing aspects of the original. The transdisciplinary increases possibilities: hybrid options might offer choices from which humans could have a lot to gain—and a lot might well be lost.

Now I'm reminded of Mike's summary of Daedalus's work and the achievement of trans-species sexuality. Maybe it wasn't just overpowering lust on the part of those ancient Greeks that had them copulating with birds and beasts. Maybe they recognized that animals have some superior aspects.

The tales of Aboriginal peoples respect animal cultures, as does using animal totems as a way of delineating the various clans. North American Indian tales are rich in stories of animal-human marriages, stories about the buffalo wife, fox woman and loon woman. These stories don't promote human dominance; they propose inter-species connectedness. There's a Cheyenne story about a girl who marries a dog by whom she has seven pups. The pups are taken away by the dog father and returned to a home in the sky where they become seven stars, the Pleiades. Human, animal and mineral worlds merge in that story.

"What are your thoughts about animal-human hybrids?" I ask Mike over a late-night glass of wine.

"I was never much interested in them."

"But you like the idea of animal clans."

"Oh, sure. And I like that song Woody Guthrie used to sing. Old Paint ..." He squints his eyes and begins to sing, loudly and not too far off key.

> When I die, take my saddle from the wall
> Put it on my old pony, and lead him from his stall
> Tie my bones to my saddle, turn our faces to the West
> And we'll ride the prairies that we love the best...

"It's a kind of a centaur image," I suggest.

"It's the animal spirit carrying on."

Mike's ideas about animals are simple and unequivocally affirmative. He likes them and he thinks they should be protected. He is a generous supporter of the SPCA and Save the Marmots, and he gives money only to panhandlers who don't have dogs out on the streets with them.

"Animals have a hard enough time without being subjected to the wretchedness of the lives of their unfortunate masters."

"What about xenotransplantation?" I ask, knowing what his response will be. "As in medical research?"

"I'm against all experimentation with animals. I don't like speciesism."

"Some of it is becoming relatively common practice. Things like the transplanting pig or cow valves into human hearts." A dear friend of ours had many extra years of life because of such pig valves, so Mike doesn't respond at once.

"They're turning humans into hybrids all the time," I continue. "There is the transplanting of baboon bone marrow for AIDS victims, and the injection of pig brain cells into the brains of people suffering from Parkinson's disease."

"I'm conflicted about these things," Mike says, "More and more, I realize that the ethical world I live in is the one of at least a century ago."

I consider raising some questions about the ethics of animal lovers who eat meat, given what we know of the slaughterhouse and the meat industry's effect on greenhouse gas emissions, but I know that meat-loving Mike will not respond positively to this line of thought. He has an admirable capacity for compartmentalization.

"I've read horrific reports," I say, "of experiments in which actual chimera are produced—they even call them that—by fusing human cells with rabbit eggs or genetically altering mice so that they can produce human sperm and eggs which could be fertilized in human beings. And about the mixing of human sperm with hamster egg cells to produce "humsters" which can then be used for a human fertility test."

"Let's talk about something else. I'm no good with change. Anyway, nothing can prepare you for real change, so there's no point thinking about it."

"Do you agree with my theory that this innovation may all be god's gentle way of helping us prepare for death by giving us a world that has become so unpalatable?"

"I won't go that far. Death would be much too much of a change for me to handle."

It's scary to think of the kind of hybrid forms that may be developed in the future, all of them serving the endless human appetite for immortality. Fundamentalists oppose the creation of hybrids, cloning, and stem cell research because they believe their religious beliefs will grant them eternal life after death. The scientists tell us that it's immoral to try to stop stem cell research because it might save human lives. But we have far too many people and they are living far too long.

I'm for a happy compromise: teach humans to forget about the afterlife and just make the best of their short lives on earth, without trying to extend it beyond its natural course. Life before death, some Unitarians say, should be our aim.

Charlotte would choose a different compromise: let's have hybrids, but let them be horses with wings, dogs with halos.

Forget about having a human presence at all. And the more I read the newspapers or watch the antics of people in large institutions or in political arenas, the more I wonder if she isn't right.

I tell her what Edward Hoagland said, "In order to really enjoy a dog, one doesn't merely try to train him to be semi-human. The point of it is to open oneself to the possibility of becoming partly a dog."

"That's very true, Nana," she acknowledges, giving me a rare nod of approval.

It would be nice to think that we could find ways of creating new and better hybrids. That there could be better humans. And maybe it's just human nature to meddle with nature. As Polixenes said to Perdita, we "mend nature" by marrying the gentle to the wild to create a normal race.

"Isn't it natural for us to want to mend nature, to make improvements in the world around us?"

You can't improve on nature. Ask your granddaughter!

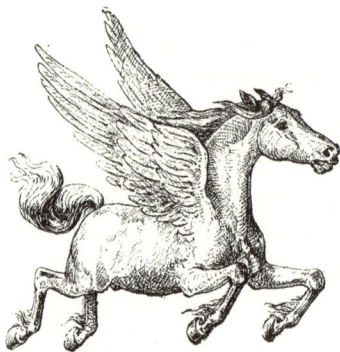

Rose

Rose died last night. As she was taking her last breaths in a Toronto hospital, I was thousands of miles away at a ballet performance. Watching the exquisite movements of the dancers, I found my thoughts were of Rose's elegant spirit, her pursuit of perfection.

When I got the message that Rose was gone, at first something in me was released and I felt grateful that she was now delivered from the pain and anxiety of her last months. But since then, my grief has been more intense than I could have expected. I doubt that even walking the labyrinth can give me solace. It is as though a door has been shut, the path has been closed off.

This morning Mike and I are walking the handsome, outdoor labyrinth with a modified Maltese pattern. Mike says this seven-circuit design feels a little incomplete. He prefers the longer distance and the many meanders of the eleven-circuit Chartres labyrinth but agrees that the octagonal design is very beautiful.

As I approach the centre, I concentrate on letting go of my grief. I gaze at the stately stone structure of one of the buildings, bright and almost shining against the autumn sky. In its high, leaded windows are reflections of clouds and above them the sky is utterly, brilliantly, blue. Although the centre of this labyrinth doesn't delineate the petals of the rose, I change positions and move to stand for a few minutes in the place where each of the six rose petals might have been and focus on their significance. *Mineral, vegetable, animal, human, angelic* realms. And then, as usual, before exiting the rose I stop at the final petal, *mystery*. Suddenly I make the connection that has always been there, Of course! At the centre of the labyrinth is a rose. Rose. And those six petals are the elements of what it is to be human, to live and to die, and to go we know not where.

But does this really answer the question of what it is to be human? These days what appears most human has to do with greed and fear. Many people I know talk nervously about the economic downturn, about how much money they've lost with the collapse of the stock market, about their worries as to whether their various pension plans will provide them with the "Freedom Fifty-Five" lifestyle they thought was their birthright. They talk about how much money they've lost in selling houses that would have been worth more later, even thought actually did make money in comparison with what they'd paid for the house. They don't mention how much wealth they must have had, must still have, in order to lose so much! Nor the astonishing good fortune of their global position which provides them with a hugely unfair proportion of the planet's wealth and resources.

Your appetites have become too large! Why do you think the Minotaur couldn't escape the labyrinth? Like the rest of you, his appetite got the best of him. He grew too big! That was his downfall. His head was enormous.

"So the labyrinth worked like a cow fence?

Cows. Bulls...

For the moment I am not concerned about the paradox of the labyrinth's design. The question I have for my guide is the invariable one: Why does it have to end like this? How can I prepare?

You know the story of Hecate. When her daughter, Demeter, raced wildly around the world searching for Persephone, it was she, Hecate, who stayed where she was, at the intersection of the two worlds, and it was she who heard Persephone's screams from the underworld where Hades had taken her. It was the wisdom of that old woman, the old crone, that allowed Demeter to save the young girl, the granddaughter.

"What does that have to do with how things end up? I don't see the point."

The point? There is no point. It's a continuous line. Things don't ever really end. Hecate, Demeter, and Persephone make up one being. A triple goddess, a generational spiral. Sometimes Persephone is represented in stories as the green corn, the new beginning, while Demeter is the gold corn of maturity and Hecate is the black corn which represents the seeds for the future. The eternal cycle. Your granddaughter is your Persephone. Your future.

"And if you have no children, no grandchildren?" I'm thinking of Rose.

It doesn't matter. The cycles will continue. Even if humans manage to destroy their own lives and the lives of other species, Gaia,

Mother Earth, whatever you want to call her, will continue. The universe will continue. Life will go on.

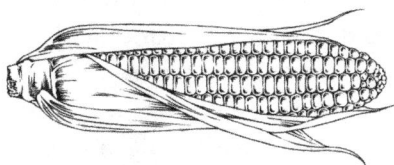

Day of the Dead

The Day of the Dead is an occasion on which spirits are believed to return to visit with family and friends. It's also All Saint's Day, originally the feast of all martyrs, a time for celebrating all the saints, known and unknown. I mark the day by going to walk a small labyrinth which was painted on what was once the parking lot for the church. I don't entirely like the feel of pavement underfoot, but I like the treed setting and the sense of the water beyond.

I'm not getting any closer to achieving the "new rooting in self," which is the goal of Jung's fifth stage of successful aging. Since Rose died, it feels as though part of me went with her. I have an intense sadness at unexpected moments and I think of all the things I might have said. That I wish I'd said. But perhaps all one can say is, "I love you," and those were our last words to each other.

The loss of a lifelong friend is different from any other bereavement. When a parent dies, we experience grief viscerally in a way we couldn't have anticipated. When our second parent dies, we begin to understand the real sadness of the word "orphan" and the state of un-belonging that it describes. Even if our parents weren't truly themselves in later years, their deaths are experienced as a loss of the people they once were, and we realize that nobody ever again in our lives will display such acute interest, welcome or not, in the everyday events of our life.

When a child dies, you feel a loss of future life and the world is diminished. If it should be your own child, your world shatters; life as you've known it comes to an end, and you must go either back into the past or on to some other place.

It's a different kind of loss that we feel when we're old and are mourning the death of a friend we have known through various stages of our lives. Even when that death is expected and perhaps welcome, we suffer intensely from the lack of a companion in a world that is becoming more and more foreign. In our later years, we really do become strangers in a strange land.

There's a song by Franz Tunder, a 17th century German composer, "By the Waters of Babylon," in which the grieving exiled people hang their organs and harps on willow trees. The song asks, how can we sing our songs in a strange land? That's how we feel when we are old and we lose an old friend.

In foreign territory, it helps to have fellow travelers. There are no guides for us, other than those we invent for ourselves, like my Ariadne, and the cohort companions who accompany us.

As a child I was fascinated by the story of the Spartan boy who stole a fox and hid it under his cloak. Rather than be discovered, he endured the pain of the fox chewing up his stomach. Those old Greeks, those crane dancers, had iron discipline; they steeled themselves to endure great pain. Stoicism would certainly be a help in facing the future. "Old age is not for the faint of heart," goes the old saying, and that's an understatement. It would be better to have toughened up when I was young. Learned those Spartan practices. I'm working from a disadvantage now.

Yet Rose, late in life, learned ways of dealing with all the things she dreaded. She had always had a pathological fear of needles and said it was simply not possible for her to undergo things such as rectal examinations, but in the end she endured that and a lot more. And now, after all she suffered, she is gone.

Everything, living or dead, is a part of the universe. There's no escaping your past and your future. Infants, corpses and ashes, all are a part of that whirling chaos.

Thanks, Ariadne. I suppose I should find that reassuring.

I don't understand why you should feel reassured. I would think it might make you feel claustrophobic, given your inclination to bolt. To make a break for it, as you say.

But it does suggest that we carry on, just in another form. It's a continuing journey. I find that heartening.

Ariadne gives me a pitying look. *It's only what it has been, in the beginning and the ending. Alpha and Omega:*

Why, all the Saints and Sages who discuss'd
Of the Two Worlds so wisely—they are thrust
Like foolish Prophets forth; their Words to Scorn
Are scatter'd, and their Mouths are stopt with Dust.

67

I'm surprised that you're familiar with *The Rubaiyat*. That's long after your time.

Goddesses don't really have a time. We live in every where and every when. Your man FitzGerald, the British translator, was a bit of a late-comer, but Omar Khayyam, the poet, was not so very far away from me in time or place. His thinking was not unlike that of my husband:

> *A loaf of Bread beneath the Bough,*
> *A Flask of Wine, a Book of Verse—and Thou*
> *Beside me singing in the Wilderness—*
> *And Wilderness is Paradise enow.*

Dionysus said something much like that when he first discovered me on Naxos.

Khayyam also says, *I came out by the same door where in I went,* which is rather like a labyrinth. Maybe there were labyrinths in Persia at that time.

Maybe . . . anything. Labyrinths have been all over the world for many centuries, but don't be maudlin, dear girl. Maybe the universe is like a labyrinth, but within that universe your one precious, individual life is indistinguishable from any other. From the time when, as your mother used to say, you were just a gleam in your father's eye, when you were a mere infant, a toddler, a child, a teenager, a young mother—at every moment until now, everything you have encountered, or done, or said, or thought, is a part of the universe. Even, I, a figment of your imagination, am a part of it all.

I tried to remind Rose that matter can't be created or destroyed, that the Law of Conservation of Energy shows us that our lives do not just disappear when we die. Leaves dropping from trees and returning to their roots. The continuation of the seasons. The possibility that maybe our own small lives are being watched or read in a distant galaxy.

And what did Rose say?

Nothing. She just looked...oh, tolerant, I guess. Thoughtful. Maybe a little cynical.

An intelligent woman. Why should she be comforted by becoming a part of the swirling, seething, sweep of the universe? If that makes you feel better about death, fine. But I really don't see why it should.

She turns away and is gone. I stay for awhile, taking pleasure in the reflective space that the people at the church have created in this labyrinth. The congregation here is a progressive one which has a broad definition of spirituality and invites critical thinking about religion. Within the old church the pews have been replaced with comfortable chairs. Now the pews, after being "winterized" with a thorough varnishing, have been placed at intervals around the perimeter of the labyrinth, which gives a lovely sense of enclosure and also offers a comfortable place to stop and contemplate before and after walking. I sit silently, trying to apply critical thought to Ariadne's words about death. They aren't much help.

Not long ago, on a Sunday drive, Mike and I discovered a newly created labyrinth in a park. A classical seven-circuit labyrinth constructed of crushed granite and paving stones in a very lovely setting, it featured a large garden with shrubs, trees, a classical knot garden and a woodland garden. Surely this is a tranquil addition to the local community which had lately been featured in the news for an increasing number of gangland shootings.

The park was busily occupied by people of all ages. An elderly couple shuffled by slowly, steering clear of the cyclists that careened through the paths. There were strolling teenagers and racing rollerbladers and the trees were full of children. A young man sat at a bench watching his daughter run around the labyrinth path, bolting past me in what seems to be a race against time.

In the surrounding garden there was one tall tree that stood apart from others. It looked vulnerable, in danger of toppling over. The tall poppy syndrome came to my mind, bringing with it thoughts of Rose and her pursuit of perfection. There was so much more I would have liked to have learned from her, and I'm filled with regret for the sad waste of time. Regret, regress. I go over the same ground in my mind and under my feet in my endless walking of labyrinths.

Mike moved briskly in and out of the center. He's proud of his speed, boasting that he can "do" an eleven-circuit Chartres-style labyrinth in precisely eleven minutes. My own progress is slow. The little girl who sped past me at the entrance was already on her way out. "This is very hard, but I can do it," she shouted to her father.

My sentiments. But, can I?

You will do it. Just as your friend Rose has done. There is no other way.

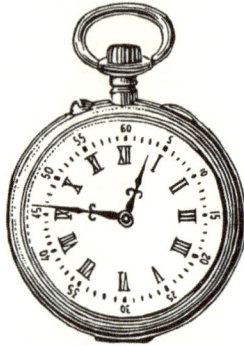

The Meaning of Life

It's time to consider one of Jung's most challenging tasks of aging: understanding the meaning of life. Is it all about love? That's what Rose would have said. Many people think the labyrinth is all about love. New-agers, having abandoned religion but still hungering for ceremony, see it as representing a non-denominational spirituality that has love at its centre. Some of the old turf labyrinths featured May Day celebrations in which a maiden waited at the centre labyrinth while aspiring young men raced through the labyrinth to win her attentions. And, of course, the crane dance was also performed in the labyrinth as a courtship ritual.

As your friend Rose and my friend Aphrodite both knew, love is important. There is always someone to love. I was happily in love with Theseus when he first came to the labyrinth. Then, after Theseus abandoned me, Dionysus, my immortal lover, came along, and I returned his passion.

Ariadne has joined me again, and she has a lovely bright aura about her that makes me think of the crown of stars that was Dionysus' first gift to her.

Love the one you're with. There's a song about that.

You have many melodies, yet you know nothing more about love than did we in ancient times. Love is old, love is new, as another of your songs claims, Love is all, love is you...

That was one of the all-time greats. But you haven't answered my question.

Love was a very big part of our lives. Indeed, we Greeks had four different words for love: eros, agapē, philia, and storgē. How could you begin to understand anything about love if you have only one word to describe it? What I felt for Theseus was eros, sensual love, but with Dionysus I experienced not only eros, but also agapē, an outpouring of love, as well as philia, which is friendship. Those would probably be close to the three kinds of love that your friend Rose was describing.

And storgē?

That's different again. It refers to the love and affection we felt for our children.

71

Her classification is not so very different from the theory of love that Rose told me about before she died, but Rose would have seen the love for children as belonging to a completely different realm, one which she didn't inhabit.

I've told you that Dionysus gave me a gift of a golden crown studded with gems and when I died, he flung it into the night sky, where it remains to this day. Corona Borealis. Now that's passion! That was eros and also agapē. Of course, he was a god, and such things were easy for him. We had a wonderful life together, and I have no regrets about it whatsoever.

I don't have many regrets about the life Rose lived; she did most of the things she'd wanted to do—traveled the world, had a successful career, enjoyed an abundance of love and friendship. She just wanted more time to do more of all those things. And she did know a lot about love. It saddens me that she will never write the book to pass on her thoughts about it.

Perhaps she's already done what needed to be done. You don't always need to write everything down. You said she was a storyteller; I believe tales that are told last longer than written words.

But then nobody knows who those tales belong to.

What does that matter? People have been telling stories of love from the beginning of time, singing and acting out their tales of passion. My labyrinth was frequently the scene of courtship ritu- als. The dance that Theseus performed as he made his way out of the labyrinth was a statement of his love for me.

Another paradox. The labyrinth, vehicle for incarceration and slaughter, has also been used as a venue for lovers to proclaim their devotion, and these days that application is getting considerable attention. Many labyrinth facilitators and Bed and Breakfast oper- ators promote the labyrinth as uniquely suited to declarations of love and wedding ceremonies.

I'm beginning to see that the labyrinth can be connected with everything. In his book, *The Lost Art of Walking*, Geoff Nicholson mentions the ways in which labyrinths have been used as a spiritual exercise and, referring to the many answers that labyrinth walkers have given questions about what labyrinths are for, has asked, iron- ically, "Is there nothing a labyrinth can't do?" It seems not.

Don't spend all your time thinking about what the labyrinth can do, my friend. Think about what you can do. Seek love, not just eros but also agapē. At this time of life, agapē is the one thing you can develop that will make a difference.

When I go to see my doctor for a routine Pap test, I'm not alarmed initially when she decides to order some blood tests. She says she wants to check my blood sugar, which has been a little high, and my cholesterol level which has not. She's always very thorough. But when her office calls to set an appointment for me to discuss the results of the lab tests, I'm taken aback, and immediately I recall that the lab requisition had included that unreliable yet ominous test, the CA-125.

"The number is only slightly elevated," says my doctor, "In fact we used to consider it within the normal range." She goes on to explain that there are many factors which can affect the results of this test and she thinks there may be no cause for alarm. Nonetheless it would be best to order a pelvic ultrasound as well as a vaginal probe. Just to be sure.

It's my own fault that they don't get clear results from the pelvic ultrasound. The instructions were to empty the bladder and drink 32 ounces of water exactly one hour before the appointment, and then not to eat or drink anything or empty the bladder until after the test was conducted. I knew that precision was important, but I was constrained by a ferry schedule which required me to be on the boat at just the time when I was to be drinking and urinating. I did my best, carrying bottled water to the ferry, but the ferry was late and I got caught up in conversations and didn't get to drink the water until about 40, not 60, minutes before the appointment. And much later, when I recalculated my liquid intake, I realized that in converting milliliters to ounces I had made an error and only drunk a little over half of what was ordered. It occurs to me that I lack the administrative skills to manage a serious illness.

"I don't have a clear picture," the technician said, "but it's OK because the probe will give us more information anyway."

I asked when I would get the results and was told it would likely be the beginning of the next week. But it wasn't. The next day my doctor called and advised me that the ovaries looked clear, but there was a thickening in the endometrial lining and so she was referring me to a gynecologist.

"It could be a number of things," she said, "but we need to check it out."

This is how it goes with cancer. You get the news a little bit at a time. Probably nothing. No need to be alarmed. Should check it out. Might be a bit of a problem, but a good prognosis. All doable. Step by step. All the way to the final stages.

The gynecologist is the next step, and he too is reassuring. Yes, he recommends day surgery, but he doesn't suspect malignancy. Probably polyps, probably benign. Of course, they will follow up with a biopsy.

"So, I shouldn't worry?" "I wouldn't."

And, after all, why should he? But time is closing in on me, and I'm still looking for answers. There was said to be a labyrinth long ago at Cumae, at the entrance to the underworld where the oracle Sybil made her home. There were many Sybils, but the Roman Sybil at Cumae was famous for her prophecies, for answering mysteries and inscribing her answers on oak leaves which were scattered to the wind. When I first read about that Sybil, I thought her challenge was for us to gather and assemble those leaves, those bits and pieces, in our own lives and to remember them and discover what they mean. But I fear that the leaves are far too many, and I too old to make sense of their messages.

Thinking about the labyrinth at Cumae I'm reminded of Lawrence Durrell's early novel, *The Dark Labyrinth*. Set on the island of Crete, it describes the journey of a group of sightseers who become trapped in a newly discovered labyrinth, Cefalu. The damp tunnels lead the travellers into corridors of the mind as well as into the centre of the labyrinth itself where the roar of the Minotaur is heard. A multi-dimensional journey in which the goal is self-knowledge.

I want to see what's at the centre of every labyrinth. Of course, whatever you discover at the centre, you find that you too are there. I will have to confront the monster who seeks to destroy me and the monster that I am. Both of them must be confronted. That's as close as I can get to "the meaning of life."

Both those monsters are indeed there at the centre. But that is not all. You will discover much more.

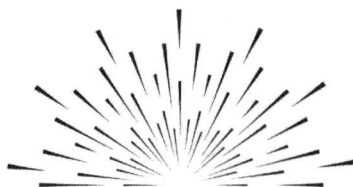

Bleak Midwinter

The end of the old year, the start of the new. We're now in the bleak midwinter and snow is falling, snow on snow. The bare branches of our huge Big Leaf maple are etched in white, and the pines and cedar branches are laden with snow turning our home into a winter wonderland, according to one of the strolling carolers who came to our house last night. Our little island is buried under a white blanket, and our golf cart cannot make it up the hills in either direction. The sense of imprisonment oppresses me, though it is cozy, even comforting, to be held here. We have food and shelter and protection from the inclement weather. So it was for the Minotaur, perhaps, dealing with the inescapability and paradox of his containment.

The white mantle around us reminds me of a labyrinth I often visited which has a welcoming space with a lovely sense of simplicity and spareness. I found the setting serene and peaceful, an ideal environment for quiet reflection, but when I first visited it, the labyrinth was incomplete and at the centre there was no defined rose, only a large empty circle of gravel. Walking alone, I experienced a profound sense of encountering absolute nothingness. Perhaps this is what I most fear. Absence. No meaning at all. The void at the end of the path. "The visible silence, still as the hourglass," to use the words of Dante Gabriel Rosetti. The endless snow, the world turning white. The last stage of successful aging is "rebirth and dying with life," but here is the simple truth: I think of death, and I am afraid. And yet it must be faced.

"But what a poor dotard must he be," said Cicero, "who has not learnt in the course of so long a life that death is not a thing to be feared? Death, that is either to be totally disregarded, if it entirely extinguishes the soul, or is even to be desired, if it brings him where he is to exist forever." This statement has a comfortable, logical grammar, but I'm neither able to desire Death, nor to disregard it. Cicero was younger than I when he made this claim. Might he not have come to think differently? In the end, surely he must have felt terror when contemplating that final extinguishing moment.

I can honestly say, though, that I sometimes welcome the idea that death is not far off. Recently my nephew emailed me a link to what he described as "an alarming flash page" at breathingearth.net. The main focus of the website is on CO_2 emissions, but it also refers to the problem of overpopulation and the fact that, at every second, three new people are born and only one dies. It has a side bar that shows a running tab on the earth's current population, and it makes me squeamish to watch the numbers shoot up from 6,774,074,331 to 6,774,074, 502 in the short time I have it on the screen.

"Look at this," I call out to Mike. "Doesn't it make you feel dizzy?"

"Why would I want to look at that?" he asks, after giving it a brief glance.

"It's horrifying, but fascinating. I can't stop looking at it."

"That seems to me very, very foolish," he says. "Turn it off right now."

"If every second, three people are born and only one dies, what do you think that says about reincarnation?" "Not enough souls to go around?"

"Yes. It explains a lot, doesn't it?"

A neighbour with a four-wheel drive truck drives us to the small passenger ferry so that we can make our way off the island, and then we travel by bus and ferry and car to get Vancouver for Christmas with Alison, Alex and Charlotte. The snow continues through Christmas Eve, Christmas Day and Boxing Day, and we are again imprisoned, but inside it is warm and the days pass easily, even throughout the Christmas morning power outage that has us sitting close to the fire, enjoying wine and cheese and crackers and discussing how we might roast the turkey over the barbecue. It is a magical moment when, suddenly, the Christmas tree lights up and the power and heat return. Our shadowy huddle is instantly transformed into cheerful festivity. We spend a lazy hour beside the tree and, from the warm interior, gaze out at the snow-clad evergreens.

Our granddaughter loves the snow. On Boxing Day, when Mike and Alex set off to try to make their way to the corner store, Charlotte calls out from the big mound of snow on which she is standing, "I'll be right here when you get back—just standing up and falling down!" and that is just what she does for a very long time. She stands up and then falls back into a snowbank, stands up and then falls down again. And again and again and again. The Sisyphisian repetition of this activity brings her only joy, not despair.

I, on the other hand, am trying to avoid falling down at all costs. I take my elegant wooden cane everywhere with me and it gives me purchase on the snowy streets.

On the last night of December, Mike and I attend an annual end-of-year labyrinth walk. There's the faintest scent of incense in the air, and a young woman plays haunting music on the oboe, a sound that enters the psyche and speaks of grief and separation. The labyrinth is more crowded than I've ever seen it, and the people are unfamiliar and various. The rosette at the centre is full of people standing or sitting in the lotus position, some with their heads bowed, some with their arms raised. A middle-aged woman dressed in layers of gypsy-like robes carries a basket of sorts. When I reach the centre, the man who has crouched on the floor in the last petal of the rosette, the one representing mystery, vacates the space, and so I occupy it for several minutes, leaving myself open to the unknown.

You know all about solving riddles, Ariadne. What's next?

The unknowable is unknowable. You must have courage, go forward, and face the unknown.

I thought your myths were supposed to help us to understand our lives.

Our stories are meant to guide your behaviour, not to give explanations. You will never make sense of Daedalus's labyrinth. It's a paradox, inescapable, impenetrable and inexplicable. How could a Minotaur be contained within that simple pattern?

The gypsy woman is now strewing rose petals along the labyrinth path. I wonder what it's supposed to symbolize. All that comes to me when I look at those wilted petals are the words *gone, gone, gone.*

You mortals worry too much. We always knew that, unless we were immortal, we must die, a fate shared with other animals. And death could happen to anyone, at any time. Young people died as often as old people; death wasn't about a lot of old people hovering on the edge of death. We all knew life couldn't last.

We didn't stay long. The music of the oboe was beautiful, but in the midst of so many people I was unable to appreciate a sense of community. I'd hoped to experience solitude and be able to settle into my own sense of loneliness. The music called for tranquil reflection, but the crowding meant brushing up against people and having to step aside in order to pass others or let them pass me. I was glad that so many people appreciated the labyrinth, but I wanted fewer of them present at the moment.

Mike says that as soon as he entered the labyrinth he wanted to shout, "OK, that's enough of the yoga and the crap, I'll give you two minutes, and then out! And the zombies and brain-deads, I want you out too. I want you all gone."

"That would have cleared the place of everyone," I tell him, "including you and me."

On New Year's Day we return and, as we enter, we hear the soothing sounds of a Bach cello suite. This, I think again, is indeed what I will want to hear as I lie dying. The young cellist is intent on his music. He plays well, and it seems wrong to be doing anything but sitting and listening. But walking in silence is another way to listen.

As I move towards the centre, the cellist shifts to the Bach Gounod *Ave Maria*. I stop to look at the south wall which has my favourite depiction of Mary Magdalen, the reproduction of Robert Lentz's painting of the dark-skinned woman, cloaked in red, who holds out the egg of generativity. The wall is covered with images of the Virgin Mary, but my favourite is this enigmatic woman with the searching eyes who gestures towards the future. I continue on my path and, as I reach the centre, the cello music changes again, this time into something modern with atonal screeches and terrifying wails. I stop and look at the row of photographs on the north wall, photographs of trees in various aspects and at different stages of their lives. Some of them appear almost human, with arms raised in celebration; others are old and tired, with amputated branches, mere stumps of what they once were. I too am experiencing a kind of amputation. Carrying on in the face of such diminishment requires more courage than I possess.

Just before Christmas, Diana sent me an email with a story about Faith, the biped dog. Born with only three legs, one of which was deformed and had to be amputated. Faith was clearly a dog with no future—his own mother tried to strangle him, and a vet recommended euthanasia—but an imaginative woman rescued him and, with bribes of peanut butter and a lot of encouragement, taught him to walk on his hind legs. It's inspiring and heartbreaking to see the little dog's courage as he trots along beside his mistress. You see him on many YouTube sites, sauntering along, hips slung forward, with the casual grace of a dancer. Fred Astaire, maybe.

His story reminds me of the lame king, whose deformity is necessary for his nobility. Maybe the amputation I'm experiencing will bring with it some new awareness, a new way of being.

Maybe...anything. There are always surprises. You think you see the whole picture, and then it all changes.

I walk slowly, wanting to think about the next steps. I am, literally, meandering, walking the winding path with its many turns. The word "meander" is a lovely one, originating from the Greek river Maiandros, famous for its many twists and turns. It is a word much loved by poets, *Five miles meandering with a mazy motion through wood and dale the sacred river ran*, Coleridge wrote of the river Alph in "Kubla Khan."

There are children playing in a corner of the room and one wild child, face painted with leaves and flowers, runs into the labyrinth, cutting across all the paths to make her way to the centre, then zig-zagging back between the walkers. I see a familiar woman, walking in her characteristic way with arms raised, palms upward. Mike said when he encountered her, he could hardly refrain from taking her aside and saying, "You just stop that right now."

Mike would always prefer the labyrinth to be empty. He wants to walk alone. I tell him that we are never and always alone, but he says that's sophistry, and perhaps he is right.

Ariadne is nowhere to be seen now. There are people ahead of me, people behind me. The cello screeches a terrible warning. I continue my journey. There is no other way.

Mike doesn't want to be alerted to bad news, but he doesn't mind passing it on to me. Yesterday he woke me up with the announcement that the stock market had dropped yet lower, there had been two more shootings in Vancouver, and that the weather forecast predicted heavy rains and northwest winds of sixty to eighty kilometers per hour. It will not be a bad thing to die and reduce the surplus population, I thought, and did not speak the words that sprang to mind: I will not be sorry when this is over.

Yet the truth is, I will. Tomorrow I will go for surgery and, although it is a straightforward procedure, I am apprehensive. I dread the anesthetic, even though it should represent an ideal death. One in which I might just fall asleep and drift away... "to cease upon the midnight with no pain."

I would rather be conscious. I want to know what I will experience at that last moment. A white light? A tunnel? Presences from the other side? A void?

Tolstoy, as he lay dying, said, "I don't understand what I'm supposed to do." It reminds me what my daughter said when, having prepared in fine detail just how to handle each moment of natural childbirth, was told she would have to have a Caesarian. "Oh, no," she said, "I haven't studied how to do a Caesarian."

There are some things for which we simply cannot prepare.

Sometimes at night when I'm half asleep I seem to feel my circulation stop for a moment. I sense death to be imminent, and my response is always to jolt awake and cry out, "No! No! No!" If I am conscious when I come up to the last moment of my life, I'm sure I will shout, "No! Wait! I need more time!" I want to watch Charlotte grow up. I want to go to her dance performances and piano recitals and see how she grows and blossoms in the years to come. I want to spend time with my lovely daughter and her fine husband. I want to watch the children of my nieces and nephews grow up and fulfill their exceptional promise—scientists, pianists, artists, veterinarians, geniuses all. I want to go with Mike to walk the labyrinths at Rheims and Amiens. In short, I'd like quite a few more meanders on this one small journey.

I'll never be ready. Like Rose, I will want more of everything. I remember that on the one occasion when Rose and I walked a labyrinth together, she turned to me at the end and said, "Can I go back in and do it again?"

Despite the winds and storms outside, I see that spring is just around the corner and just below the surface. The lilac trees have buds about to burst. The hosta shoots are pushing up from the soil. My little patch of violets is just beginning to reveal tips of tiny purple blossoms. There's a shimmer of green in the branches of trees and vines. Life abounds around me. I have books to read, things to write. Music to play, concerts to hear, plays to watch. Friends to visit, family to see. Brothers, brothers-in-law, sisters-in law. Nieces and nephews and great-nieces and great-nephews. And my friends. An unending scattering and flourishing of them. How could I leave all that?

I concentrate on what I have learned about agapē, the love which is universal and charitable. The general love for humanity. A state of joy and exultation in every aspect of creation, in each blade of grass, each leaf, each blossom. Agapē. It's a door wide open—like the English word "agape." A widespread love for the world at large. It would be a good note on which to leave.

Just let it loose. When the time comes, just let it out like a last long release of breath. Whoooooooooosssshhhhhhhhhhhhh....

Connecting

There's always something more, at least until that time when there really is nothing more. I've had another reprieve, a successful day surgery, a clear biopsy, and again I ask myself how it is that I deserve this good fortune. In no way whatsoever, that's the answer.

Yesterday, just after again receiving the all clear from my doctor, I heard a news item describing a dreadful traffic accident in Vancouver at the corner near where I lived as a child. In the years since then, I've driven past that corner hundreds of times. Now, in my mind, I place myself inside that car at that corner at that second, feel the impact of the horrendous collision. The last moment. But this is the last moment for someone else, not yet for me.

I'm lucky. I've lived almost seven decades and have escaped all the close calls, so far. After 44 years of marriage my husband and I are still not bored with each other. I have my wonderful daughter, son-in-law, granddaughter, who are the joy of my life. I have nieces and nephews and they have children, and all of them continue to surprise and delight me. A network grows before me, including the family of my son-in-law, his siblings and their offspring, all remarkable and inspiring creatures. I have my peculiar small island, good friends and a curious little dog. I've books and music, enough for several lifetimes. What is there to regret? What more to expect? It is all that could have been.

I wasn't anticipating the letter that threw me back into another life, the one that did not happen. Now I am newly connected, amazingly, with a might-have-been. Years ago, a door suddenly shut on what I had thought would be my future. Twenty years old and newly in love, I became engaged to an Estonian man and imagined a future with him that would have led me down a very different path. I think back on the time when we lived together, both studying at university, planning a shared future. I let myself drift through the possibilities of what might have been. Perhaps we would have become academics and writers, probably still living in Montreal. We would have a child who would grow up speaking Estonian and French as well as English. I would have acquired a whole new family, some in Eastern Canada, some in Europe. But one dark December night when I was away back home for a Christmas holiday with my family, Tauno shot himself, handgun to the mouth, less than six months after we'd became engaged.

For a year I was severely depressed. On the anniversary of Tauno's death, I became suicidal and was hospitalized for a brief period. As far as I could see, there was no point in living. His suicide seemed to demand my own. *Cross my heart and hope to die*, I told myself, as I imagined ways of ending my life. *Cross the street and hope to die. Cut my wrists and hope to die.*

In the end, despite feelings of guilt and betrayal, I allowed myself to live. I have read that we are intended to love deeply and then, when the time comes, to let it go. Eventually I knew I had to let that love go, and I moved on to a new life. But the old life opened up again for me as I read the letter from someone I'd heard spoken of decades ago but had never met, the daughter of Tauno's cousin.

"Allow me to introduce myself…" Julie's letter began and went on to report that Tauno's mother had died the month before. Among her papers there were letters from me. Julie said she knew I "held a special place in their hearts." I had lost contact with Tauno's parents many years before and I was touched that Reeny had cared enough to keep my letters. I was also moved by Julie's sensitivity in the way she referred to my past. "While we understand that memories are private and appreciate the personal quietness to be treasured and protected, we do want you to know that we also keep you in our thoughts," she wrote. "A chapter may close, but love is enduring. May it always be with you."

"What a gracious letter," Mike says. "You must write back immediately."

"It's so strange," I say, "to find this connection after all these years. I thought I'd reached a dead end, and now it seems as if a new way has opened up."

"Mazes have dead ends," he says, "but not labyrinths. "The maze blinds, but the labyrinth winds."

His words stay with me as I return to the labyrinth   to reflect on this new link with my past, with the wound that has not healed.

Dead ends. I have been unable to let go of the preoccupation with death, with my own dead ending.

Everything connects. If there's one thing you should have learned from our stories, that's it. You know about our hobbling dances and the geranos, the crane dance. All these dances resonated with other stories. The word for the Jewish festival of Pesach, or Passover, came from the root PSCH which means to dance with a limp. The Arabic word for "hobble" is derived from the word for partridge, which means that there are no doubt connections between our crane dance and the Arabic cock-partridge dance. The limping is a way in which we understand each other's stories.

I hop along the path, attempting to follow Ariadne's lead.

Remember what Homer wrote in the Iliad: *'Daedalus in Cnossos once contrived a dancing-floor for fair-haired Ariadne.' No mention of the Minotaur there. It's all about dancing, and a good many of the dances involve limping steps. Hobble along. You are learning about what it is to be wounded.*

Lame cranes. Wounded partridges. Hobbled old women. A nice lot of connection!

Lameness wasn't a necessarily bad thing in our time. The lameness of a king was a sacred condition. Oedipus was lame, Achilles was lame, indeed my own husband was lame. His name, Dionysus, can be translated as "The Lame God of Light," perhaps coming from Nyssa or Nyssia, the shrines where sacred lameness was cultivated.

Maybe the lame king was sacred because having a handicap made royalty somehow prosaic, something everyday.

Maybe...anything. But I was talking about the winding ways in which all our stories connect. You have something to learn from such coincidences.

Julie and I have exchanged a number of letters and emails, and this new relationship is a poignant pleasure. It has wound and bound me back into an old life that could have been, and now I am flooded with memory, awake and in dreams.

I recall a weekend when Tauno and I hitchhiked to Toronto to visit his parents. They lived in an old house in an upper floor that was not quite large enough for their heavy old-fashioned furniture and handsome, delicate china. Carrying two guitars and one beaten-up suitcase, Tauno and I arrived late at night, tired and dishevelled, and his parents received us warmly, offering baths, a comfortable bed and, in the morning, an elaborate Baltic breakfast of husky dark bread, robust cheeses, pickled fish, potato salad, hard-boiled eggs and strong coffee, followed by a strong, sweet liqueur served in beautiful tiny glasses.

I liked Tauno's parents immediately. Egon, dressed in black like Tauno, was tall and handsome with a lively, intelligent face. Reeny had curly blonde hair, bright blue eyes, scarlet lips and a wide smile, and a subtle sexiness that reminded me of the movie stars of the 1940's. The starched white blouse and straight skirt she wore showed off her slim figure. She spoke almost no English, but I loved listening to her speak her own lilting language.

I have a recurrent dream in which Tauno and I are playing our guitars and singing the folk songs of the day, the songs of Ian and Sylvia, Bob Dylan and Joan Baez. When we come to the Brothers Four song, "Greenfields," Reeny claps her hands and hums along with us. "Again," she says, in her pretty voice, "sing again."

If I'd actually had that other life, I would have come to know Julie when she was a child. I might have been close to her, as I am with my nieces and nephews. Julie has written to me about her brother's children, all of whom are pursuing artistic careers. Her oldest niece is working on her BFA and a second niece is studying acting at Sheridan College. They could have much in common with my daughter, Alison, who is just now completing an MFA in Theatre. Tauno's death was the division, the fork in the road that led away from that life to my present one, but now my correspondence with Julie is bringing those two worlds together.

"Green fields are gone now..." we sang, unaware of where things were leading. "I'll never know what made you run away," the song continued, "How can I keep searching, when dark clouds hide the way?" Perhaps it sounds trite, but that's how I felt when I learned he was dead. And here I am now, an old woman walking the labyrinth on the other side of the country, still searching.

You don't know what the final picture is until the end. When you place a new piece in the puzzle, the picture changes, and until the final piece is placed, there is always something new. The path continues to unwind.

Returning

I'm reaching the end of my exploring and beginning the return. Release, receive, return. Mike and I make a trip to see my 95-year-old uncle, my cousin and her family, and then going on to visit a niece and great-niece. That means two three-generational family visits.

On the way out of town we stop for lunch at the home of Anne and Bill Godden. Bill had just finished making his 905th finger labyrinth and said he wanted to find good homes for some of the larger wall-sized ones. I agreed to take a few to deliver to any labyrinths we visited on our travels. In the end, he convinced us to take three large labyrinths as well as a box full of small ones.

"If you go to some retreat centres, you can give them one of the wall-sized labyrinths, and you can use the others yourself when you give workshops."

Bill's collection is remarkable and various. He shows us one of his favourite constructions, a finger labyrinth patterned after the famous Versailles labyrinth constructed in 1674. At its centre is a stone that he and his wife, Anne, had brought back from a visit to the Valley of Kings on a recent trip to Egypt. Anne shares Bill's fascination with the labyrinth and has created a remarkable work of her own, an exquisite 15-inch Chartres-style needlework labyrinth with a border design that Bill helped to create based on a Greek key symbol.

I feel like Johnny Appleseed, traveling from labyrinth to labyrinth with our car filled with finger labyrinths. The director of a retreat centre we admired was delighted with hers, a large, Cretan creation formed with very small wooden strips forming the spiraling path. We agree that it looks very fine against the red bricks of the tall fireplace.

Once again, Mike and I glory in the tranquility of the countryside, the sweep of wildflowers and deep blue of the lake with its one small, rocky island just beyond the shore. It's good to walk a familiar labyrinth, the dry earth underneath, the puffs of cloud in the blue sky, the sloping path leading into the round centre with its hundreds of light and dark brown cherry pits forming an attractive mosaic pattern around the stones and symbols that visitors have left. Apparently, some people bring gifts to the labyrinth, and some take gifts away.

The cherry pits at the centre start me thinking about the word *pith*. Quintessence, crux, kernel, core. The pith is the spirit and soul of our being.

It's connected to our pithos, which is what we called the rounded vessels from Knossos. Some of them are decorated with scenes from my life, some with pictures of our labyrinth.

I'm startled to see Ariadne in this setting, but she looks very much at home, her bare feet white against the dusty path and her curly blond tresses blowing in the gentle breeze.

I've seen photographs of those pots. Pithos.

They've been around for a long time. We kept olive oil and grain and seeds in them. Essential belongings.

My uncle is still very alert, quick-witted, and full of pithy stories about family history.

"We didn't have much back then," he says, "but we had a lot of fun." He tells us about the surprise parties which took place every two or three weeks.

"You'd be sitting around the table by the light of the kerosene lamp, thinking maybe it was time to hit the sack, when there'd be a knock at the door and when you answered it you'd find fifteen or twenty people shouting, 'Surprise!' They'd have brought a bunch of sandwiches and a cake, and we'd roll up the carpet and move the furniture to the walls and have a party. One of the girls would play the piano and we'd sing and dance until two in the morning."

My uncle always did like a singsong, and he still remembers all the words to the songs of the day.

"Your mother had such a pretty voice," he says. "One year she was chosen to sing with a choir at a big concert. My mother sewed her a dress for the concert. She made it of red taffeta." His eyes have a faraway look, and I too am imagining how my mother would have looked, dark, slim and lovely in her gleaming red dress. "I thought she was the most beautiful thing I'd ever seen in my entire life."

I reach out to take his hand, but the story has made him pensive, and he turns away.

"I never imagined that I would outlive them all. I don't know what the point is in living so long. If my daughter wasn't looking after me, I'd be dead by now."

"You have a while to go," I say. "You should shoot for one hundred."

"Why the hell would I want to do that?"

Since I don't have an easy answer, we are both silent, and then he gives me a level stare.

"Sometimes," he says, "I just feel like getting up and running and running and running."

Before going on to visit our niece, we seek out a new labyrinth that has been painted on the floor of a small church. Mike wants to stop and see it as he has a particular fondness for the painted labyrinths.

"I like them because the shape and turns are so exact. They're easy to walk so you can just stay in your head the whole time."

That's the place where he likes to be. And, happily, he finds himself alone in the large hall, and he races back and forth, in and out in record time.

The volunteers at the church office are thrilled to receive Bill Godden's wall labyrinth. They gather around looking at the two possible labyrinths and choose the large wooden one with a square medieval design. The circular design edged in marbles will go to the Naramata Centre.

We go on to stop in Kelowna to visit with our niece, Nancy, and her daughter Mariah, a pretty and vivacious 11-year-old who is bursting with activity, showing us her various dance activities and telling us about the world as she finds it. It's not easy to be a single parent, but Nancy has created a comfortable home and raised a happy and capable child. I look out at the cherry tree in the back yard, profuse with ripe fruit, and think about how life goes on, despite the blocks that are encountered. Even if the journey sometimes takes us to a maze, rather than a labyrinth, one finds a way through. I look at Mariah and think again about the word "pith," and of those Greek vessels that contain essential spirits.

After stopping at a number of vineyards to taste and purchase wine, we drive on past Penticton and along the road to Naramata.

"Do you know the old Persian story of how the town of Nara-mata got its name?" Mike asks. "About the early settler who lived here, a grape grower who was renowned for his wine?"

"I do not."

"Well, apparently he was a bit of a drunkard, not always easy to understand, and when he was asked the secret of how he made such excellent wine and he replied, 'Naaaa...rrrrrrrmaaaaattttterrrrrrr, Naaaa...rrrrrrrmaaaaattttterrrrrrr, Naaaa...rrrrrrrmaaaaattttterrrrrrr.'"

"And what's that supposed to mean?"

"'No matter.' That's what he was saying. 'No matter.' It was a mystery, you see. Inexplicable. That's what he meant."

"Your capacity for inventing exotic etymologies is endless."

"I prefer them to the more conventional interpretations."

It's late when we arrive at Centre, and so we wait until morning to walk over to the outdoor labyrinth which is situated between a healing garden and a cherry orchard. As far as I can see, this labyrinth with its complex Chartres-style design has everything: a comfortable gravel path edged with green grass borders, a spacious and well-defined rose, and the traditional lunations bordering the exterior of the labyrinth.

"It doesn't have clearly-marked labyrs," Mike observes, but then agrees that, although not as clearly delineated as in painted labyrinths, they are indeed in place at the turns of the path.

Entering the labyrinth, we are regaled with the scent of phlox and flowering orange blossoms and we face a swath of silvery blue Russian olive trees. Ariadne strolls around the exterior, clearly pleased with what she sees.

The gods and goddesses of our day were vegetative deities. We danced the labyrinth in celebration of fertility—the fruitful earth and its productive people. That spirit is here in the olive trees, the cherry orchard, the scented flowers.

On this trip Mike and I are celebrating the fruitful earth by visiting vineyards. Following in your husband's footsteps.

Dionysus was the god who first brought us wine, certainly, and he should be acknowledged as the God of the Vine, but he was also the God of the Tree and the God of Nature. Of the eternal return.

I think about where we've been. All the places to which I had been before and have now returned. Returning is always complex and brings new perspectives on old understandings. The three R's of the labyrinth are Release, Receive, Return. In life they are often Remember, Regret, Return. And, if possible, a fourth R, Remediate. I haven't been as good a niece, nor cousin, nor aunt, as I would like to have been. But there is still some time for remediation.

At the centre of the labyrinth, I take my time and stop in each petal. At *mineral* I concentrate on the stone path and the sense of the word *pithos*. At *vegetable*, I look out to the cherry orchard and simply drink in the beauty of it. At *animal*, I think about Charlotte, who loves animals and has learned how to be half-dog. At *human*, I think about Ariadne's words. People have been capable of some good, even some great, achievements. It's possible that we can learn to take care of the green and growing world. At *angel*, I think about Tauno, Rose, my parents, Mike's parents, all the friends we knew who are now gone.

People die, my friend. It's not a bad thing. Only mortals long to live forever. We Olympians know what immortality is like. It lasts forever.

At *mystery*, I try to leave my mind open as I look over to the weeping willows and green fields beyond. It is all a mystery, the whole damn thing.

Your green fields are still here, aren't they? The green world will not disappear. Dionysus loved everything that budded, bloomed and blossomed. Whatever is green and growing belongs to him, and it continues. It returns.

I wish I could believe that, but the future looks grim. I sometimes despair.

You must stay the course, not quit it. What is important is what occurs on the other side of despair. When you go beyond.

91

Convergence

Labyrinths here, labyrinths there. Labyrinths, labyrinths everywhere, and not a guide in sight. I am leaving the labyrinth, have come to the end of my exploring, but I have not arrived where I started. Far from "knowing the place for the first time," I am profoundly unknowing of this new place in which I find myself. The world, more beautiful than ever before, is unfamiliar, and increasingly I am estranged from it.

Outside my window, an elegant blue heron keeps watch, standing on one foot, utterly still at the edge of the sea. On the other side of the window, unseen by the heron, I too stand on one foot, silently watching the second hand of the kitchen clock, grabbing the kitchen counter when the one wobbling standing leg threatens to give in.

"Stand on one leg at a time, one minute each side, and you'll be amazed how much your balance has improved in just one week," my physiotherapist says, counseling me after I sprained my intercostal muscles when I fell on the stairs to my office a few weeks ago. "Just make sure you're standing next to a table so that you have something to hold on to if you topple."

After practicing this foot feat for several months, I can now stand for a full minute without toppling, but not without wobbling. Charlotte can do it for minutes at a time, hopping from one foot to the other with complete ease. Alison has described a yoga position she thinks would be good for me: *Vriksha-asana.* It involves balancing on one foot while raising the other to touch the opposite thigh and bringing the arms up over the head and joining the palms. It looks attractive, a bit like a heron in fact, but it'll be a long while before I tackle that.

I don't like becoming unbalanced, don't like having words like "topple" and "wobble" applied to me. Nor do I like the words they use for the equipment that is recommended to help you keep your balance: rocker board, wobble board, disco cushion, bongo board, yoga balls. They all sound pornographic.

It's astonishing how difficult the physical world can become as one ages, but I am doing what I can to stay proactive and positive.

The physiotherapist asks me how my knees are when I squat, and I explain that it has actually been a long time since I've squatted. I don't squat, and I do everything I can to avoid bending.

"Do you know what George Burns said about that?" I ask, although clearly, she is far too young to have any notion of who George Burns was. "He said you know you're old when you bend down to tie your shoe and wonder if there's anything else you can do while you're down there."

Coming home on the ferry boat I sit across from an old man whose sad face is drawn in confusion and disappointment, as if wondering what had come to pass that brought him to who and where he now was. I can't help feeling sorry for him. Only a few seats away is an elderly foursome, each one of whom sports sun visors and tennis shoes. They are speaking loudly and laughing immoderately. I can't decide which fate would be the least unappealing.

As though he could read my mind, the sad old man turns to me with a wry smile, and I see something beautiful in his face. He is without persona, transparent and vulnerable as a child. I've seen that look, open and somehow innocent, on my father's face, and it gives me pause. Old age may be a time of greater consciousness.

Nonetheless, I don't like growing old, and having the world become so foreign to me. I'm not drawn to old people, and I don't like the workings of the new world. As a young woman I took pleasure in thinking that I had a solid idea of how things worked. My feeling now is that they don't work, not for me, not at all. Every day I'm thrown into a rage by the malfunction of one or more of the systems through which I must try to steer.

For example, a couple of days ago the cancer clinic called to remind me of my appointment the following day. I wasn't home but my husband knew I had other plans which did not include driving to Victoria for such an appointment. He said he didn't think I knew about the appointment but was told that I had been advised of it by email. The next day I phoned the clinic and was told by the clerk, "Oh yes, you cancelled your appointment." I explained that I had not cancelled anything because I hadn't been aware of an appointment, had never received the email I'd apparently been sent. "Oh, no, we never send out emails," she assured me, "You would have been notified by a letter." We talked back and forth for awhile about my non-receipt of the letter until she suddenly said, "Oh, now I see what's happened. No, we didn't send a letter. You see, there are two little asterisks at the top of this form." I expressed an interest in the significance of those asterisks, and ultimately gathered they had something to do with a new computer system, these asterisks indicating that letters were no longer being mailed out. We never did establish how I should have been expected to know about the appointment that had previously been made, but we did ultimately agree upon a date for a future time.

The next day I was at the bank, trying to make a deposit, and had to wait while the teller went from person to person to check on some information she needed.

"Is there some complication?" I asked. "Can't I just leave this with you?"

"No, no, it's just the convergence," she said, "I have to complete it…it won't be long," and then disappeared again.

Finally, after another fifteen minutes, I was able to nab her and ask, rather sternly, just what we were waiting for.

"It's the convergence," she said again, "we've changed our computer system with the convergence, and now the numbers of the days and the months don't add up."

If only they did not, I say to myself, but what I say to her is that I will come back later on when the computer has everything sorted out.

The word "labyrinthine" is often used in connection with confusing bureaucracies, red tape, bewildering computer processes. The systems we deal with. Sometimes they make us feel as though we are trapped in tortuous tunnels or corridors. I don't know about any actual labyrinths that are tunnels, but the sense of darkness and disorientation is appropriate.

Our brains are also like computers, but we don't use them anymore. Instead, we use computers. We are exploring all sorts of human-machine hybrids such as Computer-Brain Interface (CBIT) Technology, where scientists create communication pathways between human brains and external devices, connecting our biological wetware directly with the computer hardware. One of the most common uses of this technology is in the cochlear implant, a complex device with internal and external parts that allow sound signals to be transmitted directly to the brain, taking the place of non-working parts in the inner ear.

Recently I read that there is a soft organ near the cochlea of the ear which has to do with the spatial balance of the body and is known as the labyrinth. This organ is directly connected to the brain, eyes, and the skeletal system, and determines the motion of the human body. If damaged, the balance gets distorted so that a person may have difficulty walking, a disease known as labyrinthitis.

My great-niece has suffered from labyrinthitis as a consequence of an infection, and it was heart-breaking to witness this normally vivacious twelve-year-old become listless and disoriented. Labyrinthitis can be caused by colds, flu, allergies, tumours, traumas or alcohol abuse, many or all of which affect most of us, and we may have suffered from it, in mild form, without even knowing its name. The cause of the discomfort is that the vestibule of the labyrinth sends messages to the brain which don't match up with what the eyes see. This disconnect results in dizziness and nausea.

I've read a letter which Vermeer wrote to his old friend in which he speaks of the work of an artist, saying "If I understand my task, it is to reconcile man with surrounding reality." Maybe trying to resolve such a disconnect is the reason I walk the labyrinth. I'm suffering from a form of labyrinthitis and trying to find a way to make what I see in the world around me match up with my actual experience, with the path I have walked. I want to reconcile the world as I see it now with what has been and might have been.

Back in Vancouver, we take Charlotte to the Vancouver Art Gallery to see an exhibition of the Dutch Masters, I spend some time examining Vermeer's "The Love Letter," admiring the illuminated white hat of the servant and the yellow dress of the seated woman. Vermeer also said he was proud to have combined "a certain particularly intensive cobalt with a luminous, lemon-like yellow," and "The Love Letter" is testimony to his ability to portray those colours. It's a painting that speaks everywhere about the importance of love, which Vermeer also saw as a goal for an artist.

Charlotte is most interested in the paintings that take note of death, the vanitas compositions which feature flowers, birds, books and musical instruments, alongside an hourglass, a candle burning down or, best of all, a skull to show the ephemeral nature of life. Charlotte's beloved guinea pig died tragically a few weeks ago, and since then she has been preoccupied with death yet philosophical about it. Like most youngsters, she has a practical bent and was quickly absorbed in the rituals around digging a grave for Julia in a special corner of the back garden, adorning it with toys and ribbons and small statues. Each morning she takes some time to sit by the little grave in order to "watch Julia making nature." I think Alison has slipped some nasturtium seeds into the ground there to hasten the visibility of Julia's nature-making.

Now Charlotte draws me over to a painting in which a number of skulls and skeletal hands are arranged together on a table. "These people were all here together, talking and reading those books," she pronounces, "and now they're all dead." She peers at the painting and points to some pink peonies at the edge of the table. "They'll die too."

"That's life," I agree. "Everything dies, eventually."

"Even I will die one day." She thumps her chest and rolls her eyes at this bizarre notion.

"But not for a long time," I reassure her.

"Of course not," she laughs, "because I'm young! I'm just at the beginning of my life! But you and Nonno are very old."

Old, yes, I think, but not yet quite at the end. We are at the penultimate stage. As in the Bach Cello Suites, the penultimate movement is the one which allows for change, for a surprising shift when the last pieces of the puzzle are about to be placed and the full picture, which one has not seen until this moment, emerges. The structure is there, but there are also surprises

I wrote to Julie that I found it a strange and wonderful thing that I now have this connection with her after so many years of having known something of her family and shared with them a very deep loss. She replied that for her too it is rewarding, articulating my own view exquisitely. "There was always some kind of empty spot I could feel that needed attention or filling," she wrote, "and I feel as though by communicating, we are finding that place. I am very, very glad to be getting to know you. Sometimes there is a force, a compelling reason, that goes beyond what we know but is what we need. And I believe our being in touch is making some of the stars align more comfortably. If Tauno is in the heavens, then surely he is a star. And I have no doubt that he is, indeed, in the heavens."

Before leaving the city, Mike and I make a final trip to a church labyrinth. It's morning, there are a few people on the path, and the labyrinth feels peaceful. And piece-full, I tell myself, as I have put a lot of pieces together and am more at ease with where the path is taking me.

For the first time, I observe that in the large mural at the front of the hall the angel, clutching the white dove to her golden gown, is wide-eyed and perhaps a bit fearful. The Mary Magdalen on the south wall also looks apprehensive as she holds her precious egg. Each of them hangs on to what is treasured and will one day be lost. I too have felt that anxiety, but I'm ready to go on, to let go and follow through to the end. Mike is ahead of me on the path, making his way toward the exit where he will wait on one of the wooden pews until I join him.

A woman with a stony face stands in the petal representing the mineral world, and a waif-like creature stands in the human space, hands held out to each side, palms raised as though awaiting a gift. I know that Mike will have something to say about that. I stay on in the place of mystery until all the others have left. I am peaceful, appreciating the environment of this old church with its brick columns and high Tudor ceilings, feeling grateful for the labyrinth path and all that it holds.

But it's time to move on. I remember the words of Henry Wadsworth Longfellow that my mother often quoted when she was prodding me to "stop meandering" and "get on with it"—"Life is real! Life is earnest! and the Grave is not its goal."

I've walked this familiar path again and again, circling around all my anxieties. It seems now to be a container for all of life and death, for myth and mystery, mothers and daughters, husbands and lovers, rocks, trees, and sand, all of creation, every growing thing, each flower, fern, leaf or bud, the whole spiraling circus of it. I imagine viewing the world through a spiralometer, a device through which we might see every curving, curling gyre within the people and places of this great, green planet.

What have I learned from the time I've spent traveling the labyrinth? Three practical things: the understanding that comes from reflection, the recognition that new possibilities can astonish you, and an appreciation of immediacy. Above all, the labyrinth opens my senses to the possibility of change, of surprise. Even so late in life.

I'm beginning to understand what your story is about, Ariadne.

Despite the pictures on the old coins, the essential labyrinth would surely have involved underground passageways, Jungian corridors. It must have required a tunneling downwards, as in Durrell's *Dark Labyrinth*. An exploration of the subconscious.

Such journeys can lead to the development of new understanding.

It's an instructive story. Theseus is the Death Seeker in all of us. That's why he appears as the hero in almost all your adventure stories, facing death again and again.

He does what we all must do—face what we fear and, if we're lucky, return.

The Minotaur is the Devourer, a symbol of greed and self-centeredness. A monster that grows larger and larger in our times, an appetite we need to examine in ourselves. We must contain it or be destroyed by it.

No response from Ariadne, but I think I'm on the right track.

The golden thread that you gave to Theseus signifies Love. It's the only thing we have to hold on to throughout our lives. And you, Ariadne, represent the Soul, our constant guide. You accompany us along the circular path and teach us that we don't need to fear the journey. Each time we circle back to the beginning, we understand that the journey has been made and will be made again by every one of us.

And now what?

The hall is silent. I let my mind wander across oceans to a distant island where the sea is more blue than anywhere else in the world, where the golden hills and valleys are covered with cypresses and olive trees, where the air is filled with the scent of thyme and almonds and oranges and peach blossoms. White-robed people wander in the fields amidst strange and wonderful creatures; creatures with the body of horse and the head of a woman, or the head of a man with the body of a goat. The sun is warm. A flock of white cranes cross the sky, and in the distance, a flute plays a plaintive melody. At my feet, a once brilliant flower is about to scatter its seeds. There are always surprises and new beginnings. But we are not immortal, and death is our future. As Sophocles said, it would be better never to have been born, or else to leave this world as soon as possible, but we must face what's ahead.

Think of what it was like before the world was created. The vast void, chaos, from which came night. Or maybe it was the other way around. It was an enormous yawning until Eros came along. Suddenly there was desire, and all things sprang from that. Desire is the origin of the cosmos; love is the beginning of all life.

I focus on her words as I turn to make my way back out of the labyrinth. Of course, I would not choose to never have been born, to have been part of that enormous yawning. I would have chosen *eros*, *agapē, philia,* and *storgē*. All the loves of our life that Mike and I have enjoyed. I would have chosen to take the journey with Mike, with all its twists and turns, not knowing what I might encounter, nor where the path might lead. Still not knowing.

Come along, my friend, and trust your path. Living is for the moment, and there are secrets of life that still await you.

I will ask Mike what he thinks of this. He's the person whose thoughts I most want to hear. Long ago I told him that I'd heard one's Sufi master never actually told you that they were your teacher and Mike said, "Did it ever occur to you that maybe I am your Sufi teacher?" I shook my head. "No, I said, "that didn't occur to me."

But sometimes I wonder.

For the moment, though, I listen carefully to Ariadne's final words.

Enter the labyrinth. Face death—and forget it! If it doesn't kill you, you will return, filled with life and love. For now...for the time being...

Impermanence

What a lot of labyrinths we walked together through the years, Mike! What travels we had! You always said that labyrinth expert Kimberly Saward was my earthly connection to Ariadne, but you were my labyrinth companion. Kimberly wrote "Ariadne's Thread" and "Walk with Me" which speak to her years of experience in exploring and teaching about labyrinths. For many years, although she lives on another continent and we've never met, Kimberly and I have had a dynamic digital friendship and have corresponded often about Ariadne's story.

Ten years ago, we made a plan to meet up at The Labyrinth Society's gathering in New Mexico. We were excited to attend the gathering, visit friends in Santa Fe and afterwards to spend a few days with Kimberly and Jeff in Taos. Remember? But then you had that sudden gall bladder incident, and then another medical procedure and then, after a short hospitalization, you died. Lung cancer. And I was in shock. My world changed in a flash.

I'm reminded of Alice Walker's words: "We should learn to accept that change is truly the only thing that's going on always and learn to ride with it and enjoy it."

I'm doing my best, Mike. I keep trying to learn how to celebrate the life we had together and still finding ways of keeping some of your essence with me.

I walk the labyrinth and that helps me to reflect and remember, but the labyrinth experience does not hold the same peace for me that it once did. Part of it is the deep grief I feel because of your death. I think I'm also feeling the greater grief of all the global problems of the climate crisis, inequities, racism and violence It feels like everything is disappearing.

Kimberly also suffered a tragic loss and wrote to tell me about having to accept the unthinkable conclusion that the time had come to remove life support for her beautiful 38-year-old daughter after a tragic accident left her unconscious and unresponsive: *I feel shredded,* she says. And that's just the word to describe how I have felt since your death, Mike.

I know that loss is a necessary part of life and always with us: loss of childhood, loss of dreams, loss of friends, family, possession. Elizabeth Bishop wrote what I think is the best poem to describe loss. Entitled *One Art*, the poem proposes that "the art of losing isn't hard to master" as she lists her loss of keys, watches, houses and cities. But then, when she comes to the final stanza – "losing you (the joking voice, the gesture I love) – she notes that it may look like a disaster and says Write it!

I've tried to write it. I've written a book about my loss of you in this bereavement phase of my marriage. I've written about how writing about my loss of you helps me to accept that you're gone. I write about you in my journal.

What's more, since I lost you, I am losing more things, more often. I'm always looking for things. Things disappear.

Kimberly leads me back to the labyrinth with a suggestion about moving through grief and, in a new message, she says that she heard Ariadne's voice again:

I saw her standing in the shadows with her clew, her red thread glowing in the darkness, travelling out and away from her. I saw it weave through my own lifelong work with threads of all types, my knitting, sewing, stitching, and even the Celtic Knotwork I have felt so inexplicably drawn to recently. Oh, the image of that brilliant red thread weaving together the pieces and patches of my creativity! I heard Ariadne's voice say, 'Look to the Thread. It's the Thread and it has been all along.

I've tried to hold on to that thread but recently it has seemed to be broken. No longer a constant, continuous line but a broken thread. A disappearing path. That got me thinking about the paths of impermanent labyrinths.

There are many different kinds of temporary labyrinths. Some are sprayed on pavement with paint that lasts for only one season. Some are created on snowy fields on which the path disappears by spring. There are beach labyrinths that are washed away by the rising time. Some are made by crushed seashells or driftwood carved in the sand or shaped with crushed seashells. I have a beautiful photograph of a Cretan labyrinth which had been carved on the beach of a small island and was walked by barefoot woman and girls dressed in red. The women meandered and ran through it, splashing in the water as the tide rose and removed the pattern.

These are the kinds of labyrinths that inspire me now. Labyrinths that return to the ocean or to the seasons remind me that energy can be transformed. I wonder if the most important message of impermanent labyrinths is a reminder that everything we had in our life will ultimately disappear and yet be not lost?

Impermanence is everywhere.

That's Ariadne's voice back again and a message from Kimberly builds on that:

Ariadne knows a lot about impermanence, says Kimberly. When I asked Ariadne who she is, she agrees that she is an archetype, but not just in her best-known role as the woman behind the hero Theseus. That story is still told today, but her life went on to include becoming a wife, a goddess, a mother, and older woman. Strength and resilience marked her later life. The world sees her actions as a love story, but that is only part of the truth. She saved Theseus, whom she loved, and she also saved his companions and put an end to a murderous ritual. Ariadne did a lot of good in her world. But there were lots of changes.

I like the story of Ariadne starting out as a mortal woman in love with a human hero but then having a second life with a god. Dionysus raised her to become a goddess and gave her a crown which he set among the stars, Corona Borealis. It represents immortality and we still see it in the night sky. An image of hope amidst the darkness.

Everything is ephemeral, except for the gods, says Ariadne. We Gods are eternal, but all else has only a brief existence and is then gone to the underworld. Loss is a condition of human life. Your humanity requires you to make the most of each moment while you are alive. Accept change and take the next step. Follow the ascending spiral.

Kimberly picks up on that in her next message: *Mentally describing my grief as a spiraling process brings me back to my labyrinth experiences. What if… I find a finger labyrinth to trace and let myself re-experience the spiraling pathways so that I remember what it was like to be walking on the outer circuit of the Grace Cathedral labyrinth so many years ago, looking to the center with despair, thinking you can't get there from here. I did get there, of course. Maybe I need to make a conscious effort to visualise my grief as a labyrinth rather than a bottomless pit.*

Spirals used to inspire me. I was excited to see Fibonacci spiraling sequences in daisies and roses and pinecones. When I walked the labyrinth, I thought about the spirals that are present in shells and vines and galaxies, and I felt that the seed at the center of the labyrinth was a spiraling connection around the planet and through the universe. But it's harder for me to feel that now that I'm alone.

I want the labyrinth to make me feel I am part of something larger than myself, and that I can be of use in the brief time that is left to me. Some temporary labyrinths are organized for the purpose of providing assistance to others. One such labyrinth design was made from shoes which were later donated to a shelter for homeless people. In another, participants used cans of food to trace the winding path and, after walking the labyrinth, gathered the cans to donate them to a food bank.

Several years ago, Kimberly invited me to contribute a small piece of knitting to be connected with offerings from around the world to create a mile of knitting that would flank the path of the 17th century turf labyrinth at Saffron Walden. Some of the contributors were, like Kimberly, expert knitters, while others like me were clumsy amateurs, yet it all linked up to create a beautiful spectacle. The offerings were delivered over several months from various continents. Some of the knitters were able to be present to walk the path and some never saw it. It seemed a good example of how Ariadne's many threads are able to cross time and space, presence or absence.

That's a hopeful image, and Kimberly and I agree that, for us, hope is the key message we find in the labyrinths, whether permanent or temporary. Human hopefulness is the reason labyrinths continue to be created and walked all around our world. Whether permanent or temporary, they can offer paths of possibility; paths we are able to trust through whatever changes and challenges we must come to face. A spiral that can always ascend.

Ariadne drifts into view to offer a final pronouncement: *Everything passes, yet nothing vanishes. Galaxies appear and recede. Who knows how many parallel universes exist? Pay attention to what you have. Here. Now. Eternally.*

Dispatches From Lockdown Labyrinths

January 2021

I walk the labyrinth because it may help me to reflect on the shape and meaning of my life and to accept the realities of old age and death.

That's what I wrote ten years ago when I first started asking Ariadne questions about the labyrinth, about aging, and about-facing death.

My world has changed since your death, Mike. You were always my companion on those labyrinth paths. It's ten years since your death and I'm on a lonely expedition. I still have an occasional check-in with Ariadne, but mostly I'm asking questions of you now.

Like, where are you?

Up high in the kingdom of an old man with a long white beard in whom I do not believe.

While you're up high, why not leave the nonexistent old man and head for the Olympian fields? Hang out with Ariadne and her husband Dionysus? They're more like us. He was a shape-shifter but a generous husband like you, and she was devoted to him. Also, they drank a lot of wine. You'd have fun in their company.

It's not always easy to get there from here. The pathways here aren't unicursal like a labyrinth. They're multi-directional. Endless platforms.

More like a maze?

Much more than that. It's hard to understand from an earthly perspective.

I don't know what the after-death technology is like, but I do wish you could find your way to a Zoom platform, Mike. I'd really like to see you.

*

Since the pandemic arrived, digital adoption has taken a quantum leap. Near and far, everyone is talking about Zoom. And on Zoom. Two years ago we couldn't have imagined that schools and universities would offer classes digitally. Teachers and faculty members would not agree to use this technology, we thought. Students want to be in class and mingle with their friends. But now they're doing it.

You would have ranted about it, wouldn't you, Mike? At first. But then you would have figured out how to use Zoom, because you would have wanted to teach, no matter what it took.

Now we're all using it regularly in everyday life. We meet our children and grandchildren, attend concerts and book launches, participate in committee meetings, all on Zoom. The virtual has become the mundane. Today I heard someone talking about how "eerie" virtual memorial ceremonies are. He said it was helpful that we are developing new online rituals, but at times of loss we want to gather together. Seeing, hearing and touching each other in the real world.

Covid has altered the labyrinth world, and I'm trying to figure out what the change means. It's not easy. The other day, I googled *labyrinth* and *technology* and I found over seven million links. Lots of news from technology companies and articles about "the labyrinth of technology", but not much about what the labyrinths I walk have come to mean in a technological world.

Many scheduled labyrinth events have been cancelled. World Labyrinth Day was held digitally this year. Even though outdoor labyrinths allowed spacing and distancing, a lot of us felt apprehensive about being with large numbers of

105

people and passing so close by at points on the path. So we stayed home and walked virtual labyrinths.

Will the virtual options help? Turning to youthful wisdom, I sent our granddaughter an email asking if she thought technology offered a way of engaging with the labyrinth in the midst of Covid lockdowns. Young people don't use email much, I remembered, so I sent her a text as well. She replied:

Well, I think it's quite funny that you should ask this. Especially given that while sending me these questions, you had to use an entirely different platform to ensure I was able to receive this email. I think technology is important in everything we do. Without it, we couldn't progress as a society. I don't have any particularly compelling thoughts on how labyrinths might relate to this question, but I'm sure technology is as relevant to it as anything else.

Maybe. But how could an online labyrinth replace the physical feeling we always had when we followed the old labyrinth pathways? The sense of grounded-ness of the path itself while you are following the footsteps of those in front of you and aware of those behind you. Modern technology can't replace the feeling you have when you step through a line of cedar and pine trees and into a labyrinth in which a turf path is lined with lavender and rosemary. It's a sensory and spatial experience that can't be replicated.

I hear your booming laugh. *Haw! Haw! Haw!*

Don't talk to me about spatial experiences. That's where I live! In another space. And you know full well that you don't need to have your feet on the ground to walk a labyrinth. Even with Covid, you've had finger labyrinths on which to trace that path. Doesn't it give you comfort to think of our old friend, Bill Godden, making over 3,000 wooden finger labyrinths? He did that in his garage with the simplest of tools.

106

But Bill also travelled the world, walking real labyrinths! He loved discovering and treading those sacred paths, although he said he didn't find it a spiritual experience. But it was a real traditional labyrinth at a theological college that first interested him. Later he made finger labyrinths, only because he was such a good craftsman, and it was a good hobby. He kept making them out of generosity to offer as gifts for people.

Yes, Bill was a good craftsman and a very generous person, but it was his fascination with design that drew him to labyrinths. You remember that he was trained as a navigator during World War II, and he never lost his interest in patterns. The pattern and the metaphor. Now that he's in this new dimension he's becoming very interested in technology which is a great tool for people interested in patterns. Most of us think it will open up new pathways.

This doesn't sound like you, Mike. You're the one who told me that the internet was a fad!

Ah, but times change, Peaches. The Greeks taught us that change is the only constant in our lives. Remember Heraclitus? He said that time was like a river and that nature flows onwards with even the nature of the flow changing. We both step and do not step in the same rivers.

That's what you used to call me. Peaches. A name from the past, from the old Damon Runyan world of gangsters and gamblers.

But am I really talking to you now? Well, yes, of course I'm talking to you. I do it all the time. Talk to you. To Ariadne. To my old dog, Victor. But are you actually there? Are you answering me?

We are and are not.

That's your voice. But is it real? There is so much faux-ness in the world today. These days I puzzle a lot about what is real. Maybe your presence is a hallucination.

Reality. The immediate and the quotidian. That's what Wislawa Szymborska says about her unforgettable poem, "Reality Demands":

> *Reality demands*
> *we also state the following:*
> *life goes on.*

Reality demands that I accept your death. Accept that you're gone and my life goes on.

But are you really gone? I feel your presence close to me. So often. So immediately. Sometimes it's your voice. Sometimes I almost catch a glance of you. Often it's a kind of energy, or a feeling of warmth, as when you so often wrapped your sweater or jacket around my shoulders.

Is it real?

Ariadne's voice interrupts me: *What's real? You mortals spend too much time thinking about that. As one of the poets you so admire said, 'Humankind cannot bear too much reality.'*

December 2021

I'm an old person in a world that is new. A stranger in a strange place. Technology is changing everything.

Your world was a gentler one, I say to Ariadne. You weren't overwhelmed with social media and all its tweeting and twittering and texting and tiktok-ing. Everywhere now we're connected to artificial intelligence.

Why do you use the word 'artificial'? It's all just intelligence

You always had time to reflect on things. Now, with AI, everything moves too quickly. In your time, everything moved slowly. People can't remember what day it is and time has come unglued.

As your husband said, things change. That's always been so, in our time as well as yours. Change has always been the one constant in every universe. Heraclitus told us that everything is constantly shifting, changing and be-coming something other than what it was before.

Yes, he said we can't step in the same river twice. But we keep trying.

*

On my computer I have photos of us walking different labyrinths. I can scroll them so they repeat and repeat. I want to enter them. I look at those pictures and say aloud, We were there. Sometimes I look at them and think, We *are* there.

The past is real, as Penelope Lively so often wrote.

The other day a man on Twitter wrote that his 6-year-old daughter had asked, "What happens to time that has passed?" A good ques-tion, I thought. A physicist responded, saying that it stays where it is in space time, while we have just moved passed it. He compared it to walking down a road but being unable to go back to where we came from.

Yet. I think. We can't go back *yet*.

The older I get, the more present the past seems to me. Before the restaurant that is here now, I can see the one that was once there.

Below that newly painted and renovated house, I can see the old one where we used to live. Behind the old faces of my brothers, I see the boys that they were in their youth.

Everything is hypertext these days.

My paternal grandparents never had a telephone. They would have been mystified to see us chattering into our smart phones as we talk to people across hundreds and thousands of miles. My parents would have been astonished by the capacity of Zoom. Even for my generation, technology has made the miraculous commonplace.

Who knows?

February 2021

"We've gone straight from pandemic to apocalypse," my niece says.

"When will the locusts arrive?" asks my daughter.

It's not a joke. Last year the locusts swarmed in record numbers in parts of Africa and South Asia, destroying huge hectares of pastureland and causing increased food shortages in countries already challenged by Covid-19. People in those countries used to eat locusts which are high in protein and other nutrients but recently, despite these people desperately needing access to food, governments have advised them not to eat the locusts because the chemicals in the insecticides that are used to control the insects make them toxic.

These days, every crisis occurs within or alongside other crises. I live in a pretty comfortable part of the world, one that some people refer to as Lotus Land. But now, with the pandemic, the forest fires, the record-breaking heat from the "heat dome" which created temperatures 15 to 20 degrees above normal, we're having to face the fact that where we live is far from idyllic for a great many people for so many reasons.

What often preoccupies me when I think of the dire state of this beleaguered planet is our shameful treatment of the indigenous people on whose lands we live. But so much needs to be acknowledged and addressed, and it feels difficult within the current environment of concurrent crises. I can't get my head around it all.

You sometimes found that hard too, Mike. I remember the poem in your journal that said:

No brain at all. What a fright!
All my light-up bugs have missed their flight.
Walking darkly into dreadful night
for I've no brain at all.

*

Each year my friend and I write out our goals in a circle around a key word. My words are usually things like Truth, Clarity, Integrity, high-minded notions like that. But in 2020 I chose the word Reality.

I can't remember what prompted that choice. Maybe it was the pandemic? It's been real enough. Right now, there are so many crises within and alongside crises that it's hard to know where to begin. Too much reality. I wrote about that in my blog:

Ariadne was right to quote Eliot's reference to humankind being unable to bear much reality. Our response is always to cover up what we don't want to see. We numb ourselves to what we don't want to feel.

Everyone wants to escape to another place. Airplanes. Cruise ships. Some want to travel to the moon or to Mars. Apparently, hundreds of people have signed up with large deposits for such trips. Elon Musk says he wants us to become a multi-planet species that can establish a permanent human presence on Mars.

And thus the colonizing fervor continues. Destroy the world you live in and find a way to take possession of others.

*

During lockdowns, many of us who were reluctant to go to physical labyrinths chose instead to walk wooden or cloth or paper finger labyrinths. We also turned to online labyrinths. I tried to lead a workshop for a group of university faculty in which, on Zoom, each in our own home, we walked the beautiful virtual labyrinth made available through The Labyrinth Society.

The faculty who participated said they enjoyed the experience, but as a facilitator I was disappointed. I didn't feel the energy of a shared experience. As with much of Covid, it felt isolating.

And yet I do sometimes feel a buzz of connection on Zoom.

*

In *the charge in the global membrane,* B.W. Powe says "The current explosion of digital technology not only is changing the way we live and communicate but is rapidly and profoundly altering our brains.... Our brains are evolving right now—at a speed like never before..."

Yes, we are becoming cyborgs, merging our real selves within virtual activities. Our phones and tablets are part of who we are, and we connect comfortably with them. Smartwatches become our teachers, our doctors, our mothers, reporting how many steps we've taken, monitoring our heartrate, and telling us when we need to take a break. Technology, time and truth are strapped to the wrist.

A friend of mine, an artist who knits and sews and creates jewelry and small statues, usually works with clay and paints and paper. Real tangible creations that involve technique and touch and tools. Technology has inspired her to try new approaches and she tells me about a screen she can apply to her iPad which has "a bit of grab," she says, a "toothiness" that allows her to paint digitally, laying down colour, adding virtual water and blending, mixing paints, and choosing between a range of papers and brushes. The screen gives her iPad the familiar feel of paper and it offers her a labyrinthine exploration of possibility.

She notes that, although digital painting might not always have been considered "real" painting, it is now more widely accepted as another form of art involving similar skills—composition, sense of colour, proportion, and so on—as well as different skills in the process of execution.

It reminds me of the way people speak of the difference between photographs and paintings. When we think a photograph is very artistic, we sometimes describe it as "painterly." But why not just think of it as a beautiful photograph? Why the comparison? Both of these media involve the skills of vision, composition, and so forth.

We assume that photographs represent reality more accurately that paintings, but if the photographer employs various technologies such as cropping, adding filters, changing colour or lighting, we then consider it to be less real.

*

It's the pattern of the labyrinth that is important, you said, Mike. The design of it, not the purpose. I agree. I think it is also the way the labyrinth works as a metaphor. It's no accident that when you

Google "labyrinth" and "technology" you get so many results! Everyone needs a metaphor that captures the complexities of technology, and the labyrinth metaphor can do this.

In a paper entitled *The Irreducibility of Space: Labyrinths, Cities, Cyberspace*, Kirstin Veel explores the metaphor of the labyrinth as a way in which to "navigate" cyberspace, noting that the word "cyber" derives from the Greek *kybernan*, or coxswain: "The word itself thus harbors a notion of a mass of information that needs steering." The "information highway," she suggests, is the unicursal path, while the "web" indicates the concept of the maze, and the "network" resembles the structure of the rhizome.

These images alter my sense of the labyrinth and make me aware of its power as a metaphor. The labyrinth is not merely a container but also a guide for navigating what lies beyond.

I think of the three symbols Mike saw in the labyrinth myth and his thoughts of trans-species copulation, transcending the laws of physics in a labyrinth that is universal and yet can imprison, and the defying of gravity achieved through Icarus's wings. I think of Rose's theories about the three levels of love: delight that the person exists, then making each other happy, then the memories! Always there are so many levels, so many dimensions that can and can't be crossed.

May 2021

Humans have always been fascinated by the possibility of time travel. Madeleine L'Engle wrote about such things 50 years ago in her award-winning novel, *A Wrinkle in Time*. In it, she spoke of traveling through time with the help of a tesseract. The idea captured the imaginations of thousands of young and not-so-young readers around the world.

A tesseract is defined as a higher dimensional thing we can't see. It is a shape that inhabits not just length, width and depth, but also the fourth dimension which is time: the dimension that we can't see but is very real. One that we walk through every day of our lives.

Maybe the fourth dimension is like the theatrical concept of "the fourth wall," the imaginary wall the separates the viewer from the story or the audience from the stage. It's a threshold or boundary that is not really there, but we behave as though it is. All our world is a stage, and we are unable to see beyond it because time, the invisible fourth dimension, is our invisible wall. We can't see beyond the veil, to use the euphemistic description that is sometimes used to describe death.

I'd like to be able to travel beyond the veil. Mostly, I'd like to go backwards in time. About a hundred years ago there was a club at Oxford University called the Hysteron Proteron Club, the main purpose of which was to eat meals backwards They had "backwards days" periodically during which the morning started with bridge and dinner jackets, dinner and liqueurs and ended with porridge. That's like the stories in *Einstein's Dreams* in which time can flow backwards. We had a friend who argued that life would be better if it began in a coffin and then one grew younger and younger, becoming a youth in love, a child in a playground, a baby in a mother's arms and then, after a brief moment of being swept up into a mother's womb, and then swept back into the universe.

My dreams these days are shaped like tesseracts, Mike. All of time is there. There was that dream I had after watching *Wings of Desire*, the film we loved many years ago. I dreamt I was climbing up a long path in a glacial country that might have been Iceland. You were with me and I realized that we were on an island and that the only way off was by boat and that the boat went only to one place, a classroom. I was invited to go to that classroom and asked to bring my book on bereavement. I was ferried to the island by a mysterious boatswain and you couldn't come with me. People in the class asked me what it was like in the place where I'd been with

115

you. I said there were no words for it, but the teacher said the place was called *Geistganz*. In the dream I knew that *geist* meant spirit. In the morning I looked up *ganz* and found it meant something like who or all. So the place where you were, *geistganz*, must have been "all spirit". Heaven.

Some nights can be a hard day's work. But that's a good dream, Peaches, and Geistganz a good name for where I am now.

Today I heard someone on the radio speak about people presenting information by "sharing a digital space" and exploring ways in which our physical selves can meet our virtual selves. I didn't understand it, but it sounded hopeful. That digital space may be where I'll see you again. Meanwhile, I'll see you in my dreams.

*

I really wanna see you... I really wanna be with you ... but it takes so long...

I don't think you liked that 1970 George Harrison song, but I did. I felt it was spiritual, but I didn't take it literally. *Hare Krishna...Hallelujah...*

The final words of Leonard Cohen's beloved song are *I'll stand right here before the Lord of song / With nothing on my tongue but Hallelujah.*

That's real.

*

Metaphor is something that it both is and is not.

It is 0 1 0 1 0 1 0 1 0 1 0 1 0 1 0 1 0 1 0 1 0 1 0 1 0 1 0 1 0 1 0 1 0 1 0 1 0 1 0 1 0 1

It is 0 1 0 1 0 1 0 1 0 1 0 1 0 1 0 1 0 1 0 1 0 1 0 1 0 1 0 1 0 1
0 1 0 1

It is 0 1 0 1 0 1 0 1 0 1 0 1 0 1 0 1 0 1 0 1 0 1 0 1 0 1

It is 0 1 0 1 0 1 0 1 0 1 0 1 0 1 0 1 0 1 0 1

*

In metaphor we experience a gestalt shift from one distinct intellectual and emotional complex to another "in an instant of time." A metaphor, then, is a meta-image. It is multiply resonant, Jan Zwicky said in her thought-provoking book *Wisdom & Metaphor.*

*

Monks walking the labyrinths in those great 13th century cathedrals saw the labyrinth as a metaphor for the path to Jerusalem, as described in Hermann Kern's study *Through the Labyrinth,* in which he states that "Pilgrims allegedly shuffled over the labyrinth on their knees while singing prayers." It sounds painful, but perhaps less fraught than actually being in Jerusalem which remains a sacred city to people of many faiths and also a place of intense conflict and pain. When we visited Jerusalem years ago, I felt there were overlapping metaphors everywhere; The magnificent Islamic Dome of the Rock next to the Weeping Wall of the Jews and alongside the Christian Church of the Holy Sepulchre.

The path of the labyrinth very often leads us to paradox.

The symbol of the Geistganz world is a couple of seabirds.

You're getting more and more cryptic, Mike.

A pair o'ducks. Get it?

The labyrinth can be a metaphor for a kind of journey. People compare it to the life journey. It can be a spiritual journey towards a vision or it can be a journey of mindfulness. It can be a pathway to knowledge, like the Information Highway.

But sometimes, on what seemed to be a labyrinthine pathway, there's a sudden dead end or a roadblock. Nothing connects and we lose our bearings. The labyrinth has become a maze.

I think I need a tesseract to get out from where I am stuck. Something within which all dimensions are contained. As P.K Page wrote in her poem, The Maze

There is no returning
Beyond the sudden narrowing of the curve —
(eye of the nautilus, the ram's horn),
Memory fails me at every try.
I follow the spiralling pathway over and over, run —
Hoping to pass that place on the sharpening turn —
To grow small, then smaller, smaller still — and enter
The maze's vanishing point, a spark, extinguished.

Maybe it's good, to reach a place of becoming, smaller and smaller. A wise elder once told me that it was necessary to make oneself become very small – "like a bug" – to become a leader. An elder.

I think P.K. is right to say one is a spark when entering the maze's vanishing point, but I don't believe we are extinguished. I think the spark transcends that level, becomes a higher self. Maybe a light-up bug!

Every now and then, when I'm stuck in the maze, something transformative happens. A new idea and then everything connects. New understandings can emerge from that point of paradox where nothing makes sense. I think it was Deepak Chopra who said,

"Accepting paradox may not be the key to enlightenment, but it is a good place to start."

Wayne Dyer, in his book *Real Magic*, proposed, "We experience real magic when we transcend the paradox."

*

I turn back to Ariadne, the goddess of the labyrinth, for a different perspective. The world has changed in ways I don't understand, I tell her. I no longer recognize what is real. Every day of my life I depend on artificial intelligence. It's eerie.

Think of that old song you liked: The fundamental things remain as time goes by. It's the pattern that matters, and it's always shifting. Like a kaleidoscope. It's all just part of the vast and constantly shifting universe.

The shifting universe within which is the *metaverse,* the term that Neil Stephenson coined in his novel *Snow Crash* to describe a convergence of physical, augmented and virtual reality. Now Facebook's Mark Zuckerberg is creating such a place.

I hope some fundamental things will remain.

September 2021

Recently I attended a webinar where three very impressive biologists spoke about the lives of our trees and forests. Over 8,000 people attended that event digitally. That's an example of how the world has changed. Such moments of connection let us imagine that we might actually be able to change the world for the better.

These panelists spoke of trees as co-citizens and suggested that trees grow us. They spoke of the old memory in the old forests, noting that forests have been on the planet for 400 million years. That's long before humans, who've only been around for about three million years. Not very long. Viruses, however, have been around for about 1.5 billion years. A very ancient and enduring form of life. Where does our young species fit into all of this?

I think of P.K. Page's poem *Ecology:*

> If a boy
> Eats an apple
> because a bee
> collects nectar,
> what happens
> because a boy
> eats an apple?

It all connects, but sometimes the connections cause my head to hurt. My brain is not up to it. I think of Mike's verse and I wonder where all the little light-up bugs have gone?

Indigenous wisdom helps us to understand the ways in which everything connects. We have much to learn from it. Elders pass on tales from time immemorial and the stories they tell speak of care for the environment, truths that have been told since the beginning of time. Those stories are real.

*

A friend brought me a large volume containing writing and images of labyrinth symbols around the world collected by art historian Carl Schuster. Schuster spent years travelling the world to study and collect symbols and motifs of traditional cosmologies with considerable emphasis on their relationship to kinship and rebirth. He saw the labyrinth, a motif which has existed all over the planet for centuries, as a symbol of rebirth.

Schuster intended to publish some of his findings about the labyrinth but continued to study as he gathered new thoughts. It was his Colleague, Schuyler Camman, who ultimately gathered Schuster's manuscripts together and had the collection of 10 volumes published. At the conclusion of the labyrinth volume, like the sages of old and his mentor Coomaraswamy, Schuster's mind "continued to climb the Opus Mundi on the greatest of all quests: the spiritual ascent to find the meaning of Life, on the highest level of existence, beyond the Sky Door."

Everything I read in this impressive collection speaks to the importance of the single unbroken line and also of the three-dimensional maze designs in Leonardo da Vinci's "Concatenation" and in the "knots" spoken of by Dante and Durer.

You're right, Mike, it's all about the pattern, but these patterns are also puzzles and very hard to untangle, albeit a continuous line, once they reach higher dimensions. But it all hints at higher level of understandings and greater dimensions to be achieved. Some scientists say it's possible that the number of dimensions in this universe may very well stretch past four. The more I consider this, the more I feel that there are no boundaries, no separations. Only portals. Doorways.

Fred Wah often writes about the doorway. In his talk, *The Simple: With the Page Stretching Out from my Feet,* he explores the doorway as the site of metaphor and the imagination and asks: What if we just stand in the doorway?

You were also interested in the idea of the doorway, weren't you, Mike? You suggested that there was a doorway gremlin—maybe *l'esprit de la porte,* like *l'esprit d'escalier*—which, when you left a room, stole the memory of whatever it was that you had been going to do.

In many of my dreams I'm climbing an ancient winding path or walking a labyrinth in search of something and trying to get to the top or the center. In other dreams I'm exploring a many-faceted, multi-level stone structure and unable to find may way out. Often, I'm searching for a key that I've lost.

I never finish my search. Never find the key. I am often in doorways.

*

There is a lot of grief in the world these days. Global grief. Everywhere we are grieving over the plight of our planet, the
irreparable damage to the environment, the loss of hundreds of
species, the loss of old growth forests, the devastation of fires and
floods. We feel grief about Covid 19 and the intransigence of the
anti-vaxxers, the confrontations between the police and the pro-
testers. We mourn the disappearance of civil society, the widening
inequities and increasing racism and violence.

I feel surrounded by devastation, despair and death. But I'm trying
to think about consciousness as having existence in tiny little
points of lights. Tiny pixels. Smaller than the coronavirus.

Pixels, stars. Tiny dots of light in the infinite and vast starry sky of
all that exists.

When I go there I can feel your presence. I experience my connection with you as Dale Winslow writes in her poem *Presence:*

> Vibration, *translation*
> held moments, fluttering
> a million wings
> as time tears itself apart
> and sings electric waves
> through corporeal things
> *intimate, immediate.*
> *Migration, transformation —*
>
> The eye of one sees clearly
> the other held just so
> and inward draw of breath
> proceeds out through mouth
> opened to OM oval
> *— distant, transcendent.*

What's it like there, Mike? What's it like wherever you are?

Here is a place of all time. Like in your dream Geist ganz. The dimensions are endless for me now, and, truth be told, I'm not sorry to be out of all that two-dimensionality. Even three dimensionality... although there were good moments. It's mind over matter here.

Like that quotation you always had on your bulletin board? *He who lives in his mind alone is happy...* I was never quite sure what that meant.

The higher dimensions of consciousness are not visible, but they exist.

Do you still exist? In some form?

We're all here! In the end, all the light-up bugs arrive here.

Aha! Finally, you're answering physicist Enrico Fermi's famous question about the possibility of extra-terrestrial life: "Where is everybody?"

Yes, here we are, and the vast universes sparkle with our presence, casting a dazzling light that encompasses all the dimensions and lasts through each dark night in an endless spiral.

*

Carl Schuster found that the early patterns of the labyrinth have been all over the world for thousands of years: Africa, India, Spain, New Guinea, China, Sweden, Denmark, California, Pompei, Russia, New Zealand, France, Italy. And many other places. Imagine those ancient spirals circling our tiny globe, sending the unbroken line out into cyberspace! Spirals everywhere, just as mathematician Fibonacci pointed out.

The spiralling labyrinth path is everywhere and nowhere. It is and it isn't. Maybe it's like *heterotopia,* the term that Michel Foucault uses to describe a space that is not utopian or dystopian, neither good nor bad but *other.* A space that may be confusing but also transformative.

I keep returning to the path of the labyrinth in its various dimensions. Placing my feet on that physical path. Exploring the information highway on the screen. Being a-mazed by the World Wide Web. The digital network connecting everything.

And then I return to the earth. To the branches of the trees.

Seeing. Smelling. Touching. Linking. Feet back on the ground, sensing the mycelium underneath.

The labyrinth is more like mycelium than a rhizome, isn't it, Mike? Its endless branches and threads are reaching out in ways we could not have imagined. Some people refer to it as the Wood Wide Web.

This kind of multifaceted tool for navigation might takes us to a higher level where everything connects. A place that is so vast that we can no longer see how it functions as a container.

December 2021

It was a very white Christmas this year, at the end of 2021. And a white Boxing Day. And then more and more snow. I spent the evening reading our old journals and remembering that there have been other years where we endured substantial snowfalls.

We all talk about how strange the weather is becoming: heat domes, atmospheric rivers, water spouts, snow squalls. They sound like kitchen terms related to the devastation of the stove, the dishwasher, the refrigerator. It feels like that. The domestic centre of our homes being apart.

Yet that is not true, not for me, since whatever unimagined weather extremes are happening outdoors, I sit inside by my fire with plenty of warmth, food, heat, books and music. That's not the case for most of the planet although global devastation from extreme weather are causing widespread devastation and most of the people on this planet lack my comforts.

What can we do about it? I have been thinking about the Judaic phrase *tikkun olam* which is a concept that has to do with repairing or mending the world. I think originally it had a more spiritual significance related to the battle between good and evil and the need to collect broken shards of light.

I'm going to take the words "mend" and "repair" at their most basic meaning and try to apply them to my daily activities and my focus on the winding path.

*

I watch the sky turn reddish pink, pale orange and violet, as the day ends. It's the results of "scattering" I'm told. Small particles in the atmosphere change the direction of the light rays. Maybe each of us can act as a particle in the scattering of light. Do you remember that old song we used to sing at summer camp? *This little light of mine, I'm going to let it shine…Let it shine…let it shine…let it shine.*

*

It does feel like things are shattering and need of repair. It feels as though everything is splintering, cracking, turned upside down.

The old life is gone, its hours and days, all gone. The old days of the labyrinth were more straightforward. But there are different ways of seeing. Within the old path, the spiral continues but I just don't know where it is leading.

I tell myself that the brink of the unknown is also the edge of despair.

I used to talk about "blue sky" visioning, but now the sky is full of clouds. I tell myself that clouds are also beautiful.

I want to go beyond the little points of life and see a blaze of change. It will happen, I'm sure. Transformative change. Good change, I hope. But I keep thinking about all the things that may be breaking down: our underfunded public health sector, the economy, government programs. The arts, social services, small business, hospitality services; so many aspects of our daily life seem to be endangered.

I've been thinking about the Tower of Babel that C.S. Lewis called That Hideous strength in his space trilogy in which, yet again, the forces for good are pitted against the forces of evil. But what is the hideous strength: patriarchy? capitalism? Consumerism?

Certainly we have to face the evil we have created in producing too much stuff. When I drive by the landfill I see smoke rising from the staggering amount of rubbish and waste.

The three R's of the labyrinth – Release, Receive and Return – should be preceded with the six R's of survival which are Rethink, Reduce, Repair, Reuse, Repurpose, Recycle and, maybe most important, a 7th. Which would be Refuse. We need to refuse all the unnecessary stuff we are encouraged to buy every day.

I've read that Canada is, per capita, the world's worse waste producer and the average Canadian produces about 673 kilograms of waste, sending 510 kilograms of garbage to the landfill. We contribute daily to the greenhouse gas pollution and the ground water pollution, and we don't yet understand the problems we are creating for future generations.

The natural world is different. Nature doesn't create waste. In nature, material is broken down into nutrients to be used by other organisms. In the forest, we can sense the way in which everything connects and how all of us connect with a larger universe. Almost a hundred years ago, Emily Carr wrote about trees in her journal:

How absolutely full of truth they are, how full of reality. The juice and essence of life are in them; they teem with life, growth and expansion. They are a refuge for myriads of living things. As the breezes blow among them, they quiver, yet how still they stand developing with the universe.

Suzanne Simard's book *The Mother Tree* has caught the attention of people everywhere, talks about the ways in which a mother tree can be connected to hundreds of other trees. Through a mycorrhizal network she can share resources and information with nearby seedlings.

I don't understand the science of any of this but standing among the old growth trees at Wildwood Ecoforest I feel that with them I am, in Carr's words, developing with the universe.

January 2022

I can't now think of the labyrinth the way I did before the lockdown. It means something different to me now. I'll still walk the traditional labyrinths, indoor and outdoor that have sustained me in the past, but now I'll also envision the metaphorical labyrinths of the internet and the world wide web.

Eventually, I'll find the way to get to wherever you are. but I think it will be through the web of mycelium which will help me negotiate the dimensions I'll need to cross.

Today on the radio I heard the soaring melody of that old Irish song you liked, *Carrick Fergus:*

> *The river is wide...I cannot cross over*
> *Neither have I wings to fly*

It's difficult, but I will get there, Mike. I'll feel my way through the roots and threads that connect us.

You will, Peaches. You'll get here.

I'm finally beginning to see that everything connects, all of it, somewhere far beyond the Sky Door.

All of it!

But right now it's beyond me.

Exactly!

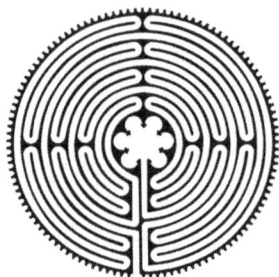

Works Consulted

Artress, Lauren. Walking a Sacred Path - Rediscovering the Labyrinth as a Spiritual Tool. New York: Riverhead Books, 1995.

Borges. Jorge Luis. Labyrinths. Penguin Books, London & New York, 1970.

Bullfinch, Thomas. Greek and Roman Mythology: The Age of Fable. New York: Dover Publications, 2000.

Calasso, Roberto. The Marriage of Cadmus and Harmony. New York:Vintage International, 1993.

Candolini, Gernot. Labyrinths: Walking Toward the Center. New York: Crossword Publishing, 2003.

Carr, Emily. Hundreds and Thousands: The Journals of Emily Carr. Douglas & McIntyre; Reprint edition, 2006.

Curry, Helen. The Way of the Labyrinth: A Powerful Meditation for Everyday Life. New York: Penguin Compass, 2000.

Durrell, Lawrence. New York. The Dark Labyrinth. E.P.Dutton & Co. 1964.

Dyer, Wayne, Real Magic: Making Miracles in All Areas of Your Life. Harper Collins, 1992.

Eliot, T.S. Four Quartets. Harcourt, 1943.

Frye, Northrop and Jay MacPherson. Biblical and Classical Myths: The Mythological Framework of Western Culture. Toronto: Univ. of Toronto Press, 2004.

Graves, Robert. The Greek Myths. Baltimore: Penguin, 1955.

Homer. The Iliad. Trans by Richmond Lattimore. Chicago: University of Chicago Press, 1951.

Hughes, Ted. <u>Birthday Letters</u>. London: Faber & Faber, 1998.

Jung, Carl. <u>Memories, Dreams and Reflections</u>. New York: Vantage Books, 1989.

Kern, Hermann. <u>Through the Labyrinth</u>. Prestel: Munich, 2000.

Kitto, H.D.F. <u>The Greeks</u>. Penguin Books. Middlesex: 1951.

Lewis, C.S. <u>A Grief Observed</u>. London: Faber and Faber, 1961

L'Engle, Madeleine. <u>A Wrinkle in Time</u>. Square Fish, 2007.

Matthews, W.H. <u>Mazes and Labyrinths - Their History & Development</u>. Longmans, Green & Co., London, 1922 - reprinted, Dover Publications, New York, 1970.

McCullough, David Wills. <u>The Unending Mystery: A Journey Through Labyrinths and Mazes</u>. New York: Pantheon Books, 2004.

Page, PK. <u>The Hidden Room: Collected poems</u>, The Pocupine's Quill, 1997.

Powe, B.W. <u>the charge in the global membrane</u>. NeoPoiesis Press, 2019.

Rayne, Aryana. <u>Labyrinths of British Columbia: A Guide for Your Journey</u>. Victoria: Labyrinth Circle Books: Somewhere on the Path Publishing, 2010.

Saward, Jeff. <u>Magical Paths - Labyrinths & Mazes in the 21st Century</u>. London: Mitchell Beazley, 2002.

Schuster, Carl. <u>Rebirth: The Labyrinth & Other Paths to Other Worlds</u>. 2018.

Senensky, Sylvia Shaindel. <u>Healing and Empowering the Feminine: A Labyrinth Journey</u>. Willmette, Illinois, Chiron Publications, 2003.

Simard, Suzanne. <u>Finding the Mother Tree: Discovering the Wisdom of the Forest</u>. Penguin Canada. 2021.

Smith, Sir William, <u>Smaller Classical Dictionary</u>. New York: E.P.Dutton, 1958.

Symborska, Wislawa. <u>New and Collected Poems</u>. Ecco, 2000.

Veel, Kristin. "<u>The Irreductability of Space</u>" <u>Labyrinths</u>, Cities, Cyberspace. The Johns Hopkins University Press, 2003.

Wah, Fred, <u>The Simple With the Page Stretching Out From My Feet</u>. Kingston, Ontario: English Department, Queen's University, 2020.

Ward, Anne G., ed. <u>The Quest for Theseus</u>. London: Pall Mall Press, 1970.

Walker, Barbara. <u>The Women's Dictionary of Symbols & Sacred Objects</u>. New York: Harper & Row, 1988.

Warner, Rex. <u>Men and Gods: Myths and Legends of the Ancient Greeks</u>. New York: New York Review Book, 2007.

Winslow, Dale. <u>Seeing the Experiment Changes it All</u>. Neo-Poiesis Press, 2021.

Zwicky, Jan. <u>Wisdom and Metaphor</u>. Gasperaus Press, 200.

Websites Consulted

Association of Universalist Women Manual: The Labyrinth www.psduua.org/auw/manual

As Time Goes By www.timegoesby.net

Breathing Earth www.breathingearth.net

Labyrinthos www.labyrinthos.net

TED talks www.ted.com

The Guardian www.guardian.co.uk/lifeandstyle/2009/apr/15

The Labyrinth Society www.labyrinthsociety.org

The Santa Rosa Labyrinth Foundation www.srlabyrinthfoundation.com

Kimberly Saward's Website www.ariadnesthread.net/

Vancouver Island Labyrinths www.vancouverislandlabyrinths.com/

Grace Cathedral www.gracecathedral.org/labyrinths/

Acknowledgments

Many people contributed to this book by stirring and encouraging my interest in labyrinths. I'm especially grateful to be able to follow and learn from Kimberly and Jeff Saward who are internationally celebrated leaders in the labyrinth world. Kimberly has been both a treasured friend and a helpful co-writer. Bill Godden was a very dear comrade whose enthusiasm for the labyrinth world was informative and exciting. Holly Carnegie Letcher continues to be an important labyrinth guide with whom it's always a pleasure to work. Members of my writing group have walked labyrinths with me and cheered me on.

Many thanks to Jay Ruzesky for publishing the first edition of Questions for Ariadne: The Labyrinth and the End of Times through Outlaw Editions and for his continued support and friendship. My publisher, Dale Winslow, has been enormously encouraging and instructive. I'm grateful to her for taking on a reworking of this book and for prompting me to write the final chapter about what might be learned from labyrinths during a time of Covid. Dale has been an inspiring friend and literary companion while designing this revised edition and has given my book a new life. I'm also very grateful to Lance Strate for his generous and thoughtful introduction which helped me to better understand what I wrote and why.

I want to thank the many people who pointed me towards labyrinth resources, shared labyrinth stories, or introduced me to labyrinths they'd created: Jean Blackburn, Darcy Dobell, Janett and Jerry Etzkorn, Lucia Gamroth, Sr. Mary Ann Gisler, Bill Godden, Lee Goode-Harris, Akira Hanson, Meg Hanson, James Hawkins, Suzanne Lamoureux, Patricia Lyster, Kim Leduc, Flo Masson, Mary Menduk, Gayla Meredith, Andrew Picton, Aryana Rayne, Sophia Rosenberg and Sheila Swanson. The labyrinth seems to awaken a spirit of sharing.

I owe a great deal to The Labyrinth Society (TLS) for the many resources the website provides. Under lockdown, I especially valued the Virtual Labyrinth Walk.

As always, I appreciate the support, encouragement and editorial assistance of all my family and friends. My daughter Alison and my niece Darcy have been particularly helpful companions in walking labyrinths with me, listening to my ideas, and offering intelligent suggestions.

CAROL MATTHEWS has been a social worker, community worker, and Dean of Human Services and Community Education at Malaspina University-College (now Vancouver Island University). She has been awarded the Association of Community Colleges National Award for Excellence in Leadership, an Honorary Doctorate of Letters Degree from Vancouver Island University, the Order of B.C., and the Queen Elizabeth II Diamond Jubilee Medal. In addition to a collection of short stories and five works of non-fiction, Carol has published short stories in a number of literary publications as well as articles in several educational journals.

Despite writing frequently about labyrinths, Carol is not a labyrinth expert but a labyrinth enthusiast who appreciates the opportunity to walk in many labyrinths and reflect on what they teach her.

Other Books by Carol Matthews

First Three Years of a Grandmother's Life

Incidental Music

Questions for Ariadne: The Labyrinth and the End of Times (1st edition)

Victor's Verses, ed.

Reflections on the C-Word: At the Centre of the Cancer Labyrinth

Dog Days (co-authored with Liza Potvin)

Minerva's Owl: The Bereavement Phase of My Marriage

CPSIA information can be obtained
at www.ICGtesting.com
Printed in the USA
BVHW040613170822
644686BV00004B/15

9 798985 833607